You may be suffering from hormone imbalance

Did you know:

- Natural hormones may reduce or even eliminate the symptoms of depression in women of all ages
- Natural hormones can banish hot flashes, night sweats, bloating, and mood swings—and make you feel sexy again
- Women who take natural hormones may experience fewer side effects than those who take their synthetic counterparts
- Natural hormones are FDA approved, yet your doctor may not know about them
- There are risks to the popular phytoestrogen alternative supplements such as black cohosh, isoflavones, soy milk, vitex, and dong quai
- Transdermal creams are the best way to absorb natural hormones
- Over-the-counter products that include the words "natural" and "progesterone" on the label may not treat your symptoms as effectively as prescription natural hormones

Learn About . . .

THE *H*ORMONE SOLUTION

"For twenty years I suffered endometriosis, chronic joint and muscle pain, irritable bladder, headaches, and other symptoms which doctors concluded were due to a neurological illness. Within four months of starting natural hormone replacement under Dr. Schwartz's care, even the worst of my symptoms eased. *The Hormone Solution* provides an enormous missing piece to the puzzle of good health. I can't imagine anyone who would not ultimately benefit from reading this book."

—A. Manette Ansay,
author of *Limbo: A Memoir* and *Vinegar Hill*

"Every woman can and will identify with this book. An immensely readable, engrossing, easy-to-read, and informative resource . . . a commonsense guide for the lay person as well as the physician."

—Maria E. Levada, M.D.,
president, Nassau County OB/GYN Society

THE
*H*ORMONE
SOLUTION

Naturally Alleviate Symptoms
of Hormone Imbalance from
Adolescence through Menopause

Erika Schwartz, M.D.

WARNER BOOKS

An AOL Time Warner Company

PUBLISHER'S NOTE: The information, advice, and program herein is not intended to replace the services of trained health professionals or be a substitute for medical advice. You are advised to consult with your health care professional with regard to matters relating to your health, and in particular regarding matters that may require diagnosis or medical attention.

Warner Books, Inc., 1271 Avenue of the Americas, New York, NY 10020
Visit our Web site at www.twbookmark.com.

An AOL Time Warner Company

Printed in the United States of America
First Printing: April 2002
10 9 8 7 6 5 4 3 2 1

Library of Congress Cataloging-in-Publication Data
Schwartz, Erika.
    The hormone solution : naturally alleviate symptoms of hormone
    imbalance from adolescence through menopause / Erika Schwartz.
        p. cm.
    Includes bibliographical references and index.
    ISBN 0-446-67828-7
        1. Hormone therapy. 2. Menopause—Hormone therapy.
    3. Menopause—Alternative treatment. 4. Middle aged women—
    Health and hygiene. I. Title.

RG186 .S39 2002
618.1'7506—dc21
                                                        2001046643

Book design and text composition by Ellen Gleeson
Cover design by Brigid Pearson

To Katie and Lisa, my guardian angels
To Ken, my love

※ ACKNOWLEDGMENTS ※

$\mathscr{I}$ hope you find this book as easy to read as it was to write. Being surrounded by good friends and knowledgeable advisers, when dealing with a topic for which everyone desperately needs information and solutions, made my work rewarding and inspiring.

Christine Iurato, my friend and partner in the development of the Hormone Solution Program. I thank you for being so generous with your time, your brilliant advice, your knowledge, your care.

Deborah Schneider, my agent, friend, and cheerleader. Thank you for leading me to natural hormones and keeping the faith in my ability to write on my own.

My friend Joe Bova, thank you for always being there to teach me the intricacies of pharmaceuticals and nutraceuticals.

Robert Giuliano, thank you for allowing me the use of your lab to work out combinations of natural hormones.

At Warner Books, my editor Diana Baroni and assistant editor Molly Chehak, your insightful guidance made my job a pleasure. Thank you for your patience.

Thank you to my patients. You are my source of strength, information, and faith. Your stories will undoubtedly help improve the lives of many.

CONTENTS

✤ AUTHOR'S NOTE ✤

*T*he program described in this book is not intended to be a substitute for medical care and advice. You are advised to consult with your health care professional with regard to all matters relating to your health, including matters that may require diagnosis or medical attention. In particular, if you have any special condition requiring medical attention, or if you are taking or have been advised to take (or to refrain from taking) any medication, you should consult regularly with your physician.

The identity of some of the patients referred to in this book, and certain details about them, have been modified or are presented in composite form.

The information provided in this book is based on sources that the author believes to be reliable, and information regarding products and companies is current as of December 2001.

*A*lmost twenty years ago, I opened my first private practice—an outfit so small that it fit into a garage in Westchester County. Prior to that, I had done my residency at Kings County Hospital Center, the second largest hospital in the country, and was director of the Emergency Department at Westchester County Medical Center in Valhalla, New York. While my years at the medical center were exciting and action packed, I began to feel that I was missing the extended, close patient contact I knew private practice could offer. I wanted to be part of my patients' everyday lives and have a role in keeping them well. Over the years, my practice grew and began to reflect my philosophy that the absence of disease does *not* equal wellness. *Being well* means *feeling* well, and feeling well definitely does not include constantly worrying about being sick.

The more I practiced medicine, the more I focused on finding the source of this fear and worry, eliminating the possibility of disease, and then looking for ways to treat the root cause. Women of all ages came to me with the same issue: They looked healthy, their test results came back normal, yet they *felt* miserable. The more experienced I became, the more I realized that hormones were the common thread in all of these women's situations. In addition, I, too, experienced the debilitating effects of hormone imbalance. I had been through depression before my periods, incapacitating cramps and migraines when taking birth control pills, night sweats after the birth of my first daughter, loss of sex drive after the birth of both daughters. I worried every month when I felt lumps in my breasts before my period. I was sure they were breast cancer and I'd never live to see my kids grow up. Needless to say, I worried a lot. I was lucky, though, because being a doctor forced me to learn to deal with the worry, and gave me the opportunity to help other women deal with it as well.

Hormone changes, imbalances, and deficiencies turned out to be the root cause of many of my patients' (and my own) health problems. I struggled to find solutions for young girls with mood swings and depression and young women with postpartum depression, PMS, PMDD, migraines, and fertility problems. I relied on conventional therapies to treat women in their middle years for menopausal symptoms, the mainstays of which still were synthetic estrogens and progestins. Some patients took birth control pills to stave off the symptoms of menopause; others took Premarin and Provera. These methods never seemed to work, as my patients would continually return to my office complaining of symptoms. If the hot flashes disappeared, the trade-off was sore, swollen breasts and return of never-ending, heavy periods. If the period was gone, headaches and migraines overwhelmed the women. My patients were unhappy and so was I, as their doctor. At that time, I still believed standard conventional hormone replacement therapy was the only option. After all, most of my colleagues used it and felt it offered reasonable results.

But then it happened to me: At forty-six years old, I went through The Change myself. I began to wake up in a pool of perspiration, my heart pounding so hard I thought I was having a heart attack. I could no longer sleep. With my long work hours, the sight of a bed used to be enough to make me fall asleep. Yet suddenly, sleep had become my enemy. And that was only one of many strange symptoms I was experiencing. My weight had never been a problem in my twenties and thirties. Then gradually, over a six-year span after I turned forty, I gained 15 pounds. I worked out regularly and ate a healthy diet. Yet, somehow, I could not shed the weight. *Frustration* became part of my emotional vocabulary. My joints hurt, my hair was thinning, I felt drained.

I too embarked on a program of standard hormone replacement therapy but felt increasingly miserable with every passing day. My breasts were swollen balloons and my period, once gone, returned with a vengeance not once a month, but rather two and three times. My moods had never been a serious issue, but on conventional hormone replacement I became a stranger to myself. One moment I was on top of the world; the next I was crying. And the bloating! My clothes just didn't fit, my body was changing shape, and my sex drive disappeared as my night sweats and sleep deprivation increased. Now I was complaining, too. It seemed as though nothing could help me or my patients feel normal again.

Why wasn't there a viable solution to reducing the symptoms of menopause? After ten years of practicing medicine, I found this to be ridiculous. After all, menopause is just another change in hormone balance. I became determined to find a solution. To treat the symptoms of menopause, I began to try a combination of conventional and alternative remedies and had my patients try them with me. The results were disappointing. Some medications worked for a while, some herbs and supplements alleviated some of the symptoms some of the time, while others had dangerous side effects. Some did nothing more than lighten our wallets.

The only medications that I found that consistently

worked were natural hormones. Medically supervised natural hormone treatment using estrogens and progesterone made from the synthesis of yams and soy proved nothing short of miraculous. Safe, easy to administer, and consistently effective, natural hormones worked. Creating and fine-tuning my own program for the administration of natural hormones became my mission. The patients who joined me in the use of natural hormones reported consistent improvements in all aspects of their lives. Gone were the hot flashes, the night sweats, the mood swings, the bloating. Lo and behold, even our sex drive returned! And we didn't have to put up with swollen, tender breasts or the return of the dreaded period. Above all, menopause was no longer a torture. It was just another change. I personally felt great on my own program, and, with my life back on track, I wanted to bring natural hormones to all women. Initially, I thought *all women* meant *menopausal women,* but that turned out to be far too limited. If natural hormones worked on menopausal women, why woudn't they work on young women suffering from symptoms of hormone imbalance as well?

Cautiously, I started using natural progesterone on young women. The road had been paved by work done by Drs. John Lee, Jonathan Wright, and Joel Hargrove. The results were remarkable. My patients with symptoms known to be caused by hormone imbalance felt better on the natural hormones than on more conventional medicines. From my clinical experience, I learned that symptoms believed to be limited to menopause occur throughout our lives. A flurry of women taking antidepressants joined my patient list and started taking natural hormones. Remarkably, within a few months many were able to stop taking their medications, while those who were still taking them, took less.

What I had not realized before was that all these hormone imbalances are connected and could be treated successfully with natural hormone supplementation. The more women of different ages with different symptoms came to see me, the more convinced I became of the continuum of hormone changes we are subjected to at all ages. Natural hormone treatment was invariably successful and had none of the side effects associated with other types of medications. That was because natural hormones treated the root cause of the problems with substances closely resembling the missing or out-of-balance hormones our bodies make. There were no potentially harmful, synthetic substitutes in this hormone supplementation program.

The remarkable results in my practice—and across the country in the practices of other physicians prescribing natural hormones—reinforced my belief in the efficacy of natural hormones. They represent the immediate solution we are all looking for. This book explains why your doctor may not know about them, why he or she may be reluctant to help you by prescribing them, and how to bring your doctor into the loop of this nothing-short-of-miraculous solution.

The Hormone Solution tackles this area of confusion in women's lives. The information I provide will help you take charge of your own health, giving you the knowledge you need to understand how hormone imbalance affects your everyday life and, subsequently, all the existing options for restoring balance and health. As a physician with twenty years of experience and a thriving practice specializing in hormone supplementation—and as a menopausal woman with firsthand experience with both synthetic and natural hormones—I am uniquely qualified to share my expertise and story with you. In fact, how I learned about natural hormones and came to develop a practice around them may be of particular interest to you, as many of you may see shades of yourself and your frustration in my story. My hope is that this book will help you understand the difference between synthetic and natural hormones and give you the scientific information you need to be able to distinguish between the possible dangers of synthetic hormones and the benefits of natural hormones.

A recent article titled "Hormone Therapy: Doubts Grow" (*USA Today,* June 13, 2001) brought the latest information on hormone replacement therapy, contained in the previous day's issue of the *Journal of the American Medical Association,* to millions of readers nationwide. In an already deep sea of doubt about the efficacy and long-term effects of HRT, more doubt and confusion were added by this article. According to it, "34% of middle-age women take estrogen, and progesterone, either alone or in combination." Most of these women are taking HRT hoping to prevent heart disease, osteoporosis, Alzheimer's, and other troublesome chronic illnesses associated with aging. As the article brought to light, however, many in the medical community aren't convinced that HRT actually protects from chronic illnesses, and many have fears about its association with cancer of the ovaries, the uterus, and the breasts. These doubts persist for several reasons.

Even though HRT has been around for more than thirty years, only four significant studies have been conducted to evaluate this form of therapy. The results of these studies are equivocal at best. Another limitation is that they were conducted almost exclusively on synthetic hormones. Although natural hormones are another FDA-approved form of hormones, they were not included in these studies. And to make things even more difficult, little information about them reaches physicians or the public at large.

The following chapters will give you a comprehensive overview of conventional and alternative treatments available for symptoms of hormone imbalance at any age, from your teens on up to your menopausal years. The decision to use natural hormones as part of an integrated program of diet, exercise, and lifestyle is yours and should come from a position of knowledge and strength. *The Hormone Solution* gives you all the information you need to reach this decision. And since hormone imbalance is not limited to women, men's issues are also addressed.

I have successfully implemented in my practice the program detailed in these pages—using natural hormones to correct hormone imbalance and help relieve the resulting symptoms. Read this book and see how easy it can be to make a change for the better you never thought could happen. If you are like me and the women I care for, you don't need to suffer any longer. *The Hormone Solution* can change your life.

THE
Hormone
SOLUTION

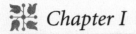

Chapter I

How Did We Get Here?

*M*enopause is not a pause. While *menopause* literally means "cessation of menstrual periods," for most women it defines the most traumatic part of their lives. It forces them to confront the inevitability of aging. It is not a glorious transition; it is not a time when women feel free and empowered.

As one of my patients put it, "The menopausal experience changes one's sense of self. Lots of little things go wrong and then suddenly, one day, you find you are not the same person anymore." It is the accumulation of many symptoms and changes that become progressively less manageable and end up all too often with disastrous consequences. These disastrous consequences affect more than forty-three million women today, along with twenty-one million women who will be reaching their menopausal years in the next decade. The research on menopause is limited, solutions scarce, information contradictory. In 1993, the National Institutes of Health started a ten-year study to compare hormone replacement therapy with diet, exercise, and calcium supplementation in the prevention of cancer, heart disease, and osteoporosis. The results of this study will not be available until 2005 at the earliest. Who has time to wait until then? Definitely not the millions of women suffering from symptoms of hormone imbalance today. Those women have options; all they need is an understanding that menopause is simply another change—it does not happen overnight—it's another transition in the continuum of change in our lives.

Indeed, long before we reach the point of being overwhelmed by the symptoms of menopause, long before we feel totally betrayed by our bodies, little by little, one symptom at a time, menopause unfolds over more than thirty years. The key to preventing the serious and devastating problems created by menopause is found in understanding the correlation between these symptoms we experience at all times during our lives and the hormone imbalance that causes them. The symptoms begin when we are in our teens, and they follow us throughout our lives with incredible tenacity. Let's look back in time and see when they begin and what causes them to occur. Once we realize that these symptoms are part of our lives at all ages, we can uncover their root cause. If we connect our symptoms to the particular type of hormone imbalance that causes them—regardless of age—then we can treat the problem and prevent it from recurring or getting worse. In *The Hormone Solution,* I'll provide you with a comprehensive solution for the treatment of the normal changes that affect women (and men) throughout their lives.

Does the following sound familiar? You're thirteen. You are an accomplished athlete and a tomboy. You refuse to wear dresses even when you go to church. Your mother is concerned because all your friends have gotten their periods while you show no signs—no breast buds, no perspiration odor, no pubic hair. Your mother takes you to the doctor, and your blood tests, physical examination, and CT brain scan are normal. Nothing changes for another three years. And then, over a period of six months, you become a girl—

you stop being a tomboy, you grow breasts, get your period, and start blushing when you meet a boy.

Or maybe this rings a bell? You're twenty-four. You just had your second child. The pregnancy was uneventful, and your baby is beautiful and healthy. Although you have plenty of support from your family and friends, you're getting depressed. With each passing day, your family helplessly watches you lose interest in the baby and yourself. You finally give in to your husband's pleas to go see a doctor. You're diagnosed with postpartum depression.

Perhaps you're at a later stage: You remember when you were thirty-two and would come home from work and finally finish with the husband, the kids, and the phone calls. Those were the days when you were done with another long but rewarding day and couldn't wait to hit the sack. You'd crawl into bed and fall asleep within a minute. You slept as if you were in a coma. Now, fifteen years later, you're forty-seven. Your job is secure, your kids have their driver's licenses and are ready to go to college, your husband and you have stopped bickering over the position of the toilet seat cover, and just when you thought things should be getting easier, something very strange has happened.

By 10 P.M., you are so exhausted you barely make it through brushing your teeth and applying your five different antiwrinkle creams guaranteed to take ten years off your face. You're extremely tired but you dread getting into bed because you know what follows will be a torture you never believed possible. And yet, you have no choice, you know you need the rest. So you go to bed, and thankfully, you fall asleep: but not for long. Suddenly, it feels as though a bolt of lightning has shot through you. You jump up, it's 2 A.M., you're lying in a pool of sweat, and your body temperature feels high enough to boil water. The sheets are twisted around you; your heart is pounding hard. You're fairly sure you aren't having a heart attack because the same thing has happened every night for months now. Suddenly, you realize you have to pee so badly that you're not sure you can make it to the bathroom. Holding on to the walls, you reach the toilet and pray this activity won't wake you up too much. You return to bed and pull the blanket to your nose as a cold shiver runs through your body. You close your eyes and try not to think of the perspiration-soaked sheets, which have now turned to ice. You look around and wonder why the man lying next to you is sleeping soundly. You lie awake for hours desperately wanting and needing to sleep. When the alarm goes off in the morning, you want to die. You cannot believe it's time to start another day feeling this way.

What happened? What has changed between the time you were thirteen and forty-seven?

The answer is simple: Your hormones. Let's assume that our lives are a jigsaw puzzle. The pieces that make up the puzzle are our hormones. Having all the pieces isn't enough. What we must know is how the pieces fit and, once they do, how to keep the puzzle together. When you're thirteen, you clearly lived in a world where the puzzle fits neatly and flawlessly. While your hormones may not follow the expected mold—breast buds at eleven, menstruation at thirteen— you're fine. Your hormones balance themselves and find the happy medium to keep you healthy and normal. At twenty-four, postpartum depression represents a common example of hormone imbalance of a more severe type. By forty-seven, the problems appear insurmountable. Our hormones, the pieces of the puzzle, begin to come apart, and we either figure out how to fit them together again, or we become sick, we feel old.

The Hormone Solution will teach you how to identify each piece of the puzzle, make the pieces fit, and give you the secret to keeping the puzzle intact for years to come. I will give you the background you need to build the foundation that keeps your body and mind in perfect balance. If you understand how your body works, you can help forestall illness, get rid of unwanted symptoms, and restore your energy and vitality.

This may sound like a tall order, but I promise you it's not. I won't waste your time with intricate, medical detail. While understanding the complex physiology of hormones may be interesting, it's their application to our personal lives that really matters.

THE HORMONE STORY

Hormones are products of living cells that circulate in our bodily fluids and produce specific effects on the activity of other cells far removed from the organs where the hormones are made. They stimulate or inhibit the actions of cells everywhere in the body. No organ is left untouched by the actions of hormones. Hormones, however, cannot be seen with the naked eye, and this situation makes them very difficult to understand.

Endocrinology: The Study of Hormones

In the 1970s, when I went to medical school, endocrinology, the medical subspecialty involved in the diagnosis and treatment of diseases of hormones and the glands that make them, was not a popular course. It was complicated, it dealt with intangibles, and few students could grasp it. Hormones were complex structures, critical to the proper function of the human body, yet impossible to pin down. Even when dealing with diseases, they were difficult to evaluate by our medical testing methods. Everywhere you turned, be it in illness or in health, you saw their effects on men and women, yet our profession could not control them.

Blood tests were inadequate and cumbersome, and no radiologic techniques for evaluating the actions of hormones existed. Testing pituitary (master gland) function was hell for both patient and physician. We tested only for disease. The tests were complicated, they took days to perform, the patients were invariably very sick, and the results were difficult to interpret. Laboratory and clinical research was intricate and laborious, and the information published in the scientific literature was mostly esoteric, pertaining mainly to animals and not humans. As a result, few medical students chose endocrinology as their career.

Even now, endocrinology, with its focus on disease—diabetes, thyroid, pituitary, and genetic hormone imbalances—is not a popular specialty. There has never been a glut of endocrinologists, which very well may be the reason why the study of hormones and how to balance them has become an area for wellness experts and anti-aging specialists.

The Importance of Hormones

Hormones run through our bodies with great speed. They have the power to make us feel well, but they can also wreck our lives. There are many types of hormones, all with important roles in keeping us balanced and healthy. They balance our sugar level, instruct our cells to generate energy, keep our calcium level normal and our hearts beating regularly, and help our liver detoxify our system even after a five-martini night. Even with twenty-six years of clinical medical experience and my present focus on the study of hormones, I am still utterly fascinated by their impact on the human body. Although there are a lot of known hormones controlling our body's functions, I believe one particular hormone group reigns supreme: the sex hormones. These are estrogen, progesterone, and testosterone. They determine our gender; they are responsible for our outlook on and reactions to life, how we age, and ultimately how long we live.

The Primitive Master Gland: The Hypothalamus

Hormones are produced by lots of organs, but their production and actions are always rigidly controlled by the master gland—the hypothalamus (hi-po-THA-la-mus, a pinhead structure buried in the middle of the brain, above the pituitary gland). The hypothalamus literally supervises the synchronization of hormone release. We don't know how the hypothalamus got to be in charge of all hormone balance. Its mysterious function has been studied for many years. The most commonly accepted belief is that the hypothalamus is a very old organ linked to early animal evolution; it was allegedly there before the pituitary existed and before sexes were differentiated. Its role was to control basic body functions—heartbeat, breathing, digestion, reproduction, excretion. Throughout evolution, the hypothalamus has maintained its controlling role by making the one hormone that coordinates all sex hormones: *gonadotropin-releasing hormone (GnRH)*.

Through a system of blood vessels inside the brain, this hormone goes directly to the pituitary and stimulates it to release its own set of hormones with the final role of modulating end-organ sexual hormone production. "End organ" refers to the ovaries, testes, and adrenal glands; the hormones they produce are estrogen, progesterone, and testosterone, among others. Remarkably, this one hormone (GnRH) monitors the production and effects of hormones made by the pituitary, the ovaries or testes, and the adrenals. This remarkable feat is the main reason why the hypothalamus is one of the key pieces in the hormone puzzle.

Along the evolutionary ladder, a new organ developed between the hypothalamus and the other organs (heart, lungs, stomach, ovaries, testes, adrenals). That organ is the pituitary.

The Modern Master Gland: The Pituitary

Below the hypothalamus, buried in the middle of the brain, lies the pituitary gland. While we consider the hypothalamus a primitive, old remnant of an antique glandular system, the pituitary is much newer—the modern-age master gland. Arbitrarily divided by physiologists into anterior and posterior portions, the pituitary produces a lot of different hormones. All sex-hormone-releasing and -inhibiting factors are produced by the anterior portion of the pituitary gland. It is there, in an area of a few millimeters, that the headquarters of hormone regulation are located.

The anterior pituitary is in charge of stimulating or blocking the release of the principal sex hormones— estrogen, progesterone, and testosterone. This is accomplished through the actions of two hormones secreted by the anterior pituitary: *follicle-stimulating hormone (FSH)* and *luteinizing hormone (LH)*. FSH and LH are directly responsible for cycling the production of estrogen and progesterone by the organs that produce them (ovaries, adrenals, and corpus luteum). FSH stimulates estrogen production, while LH stimulates progesterone production. FSH and LH work together to balance estrogen and progesterone levels. Another sex-related hormone produced by the pituitary, *prolactin* is released primarily after a woman gives birth. Its role is to stimulate the breast to produce milk and to shrink the size of the uterus back to normal.

How Do FSH and LH Work?

Let's take an average twenty-eight-day menstrual cycle, when you aren't pregnant. We'll start with day 1. You have just started your period. Your estrogen and progesterone levels are practically nil. The lack of hormones in your system is what has induced you to get your period.

GnRH from the hypothalamus and FSH from the pituitary are excreted in response to the level of estrogen circulating in your bloodstream. On day 1, as the blood washes against the hypothalamus and anterior pituitary, there's practically no estrogen in it. The hypothalamus thus sends out its hormone GnRH to wake up the pituitary. The receptors on the cells that make up the anterior pituitary gland respond to the rise in GnRH and the lack of estrogen in the bloodstream. Their response is to release FSH into the bloodstream. The presence of FSH stimulates the ovaries and adrenals to start making estrogen. For the following ten days of the normal cycle, the anterior pituitary gland will be pouring out FSH to stimulate the ovaries to make estrogen.

Indirectly, the high levels of FSH—together with the now-rising levels of estrogen—are responsible for another important job. Remember that *FSH* stands for "follicle-stimulating hormone." Its job is to stimulate the formation of the follicle and the maturation of an egg. In one of the ovaries, an egg has been identified. This egg (ovum) will become mature over the following ten days. It is this egg that will be expelled from the ovary at the time of ovulation, fifteen days before the end of the cycle. If fertilized by a sperm, this is the egg that will become a baby nine months later.

FSH and estrogen prepare the egg for ovulation. This part of the cycle is called the *follicular phase*. It is during this phase that the ovaries are making estrogen and testosterone to help the egg ripen. As it ripens, the egg is surrounded by a protective bubble, the follicle, which develops as the egg matures. Once mature, the egg is expelled from the ovary on ovulation day. The follicle is left behind in the ovary and it becomes the corpus luteum, which produces progesterone.

As this scenario unfolds, the increased levels of estrogen produced by the ovaries and follicle are now reaching the pituitary and sending a new message to the master gland: "We have enough estrogen here to go ahead and ovulate."

If the pituitary reads the message correctly, it starts releasing LH (luteinizing hormone). LH promotes ovulation. Within ten to twelve hours of the spike of LH in your bloodstream, you ovulate. LH stimulates the production of progesterone, the thinning of the wall of the ovary, the expulsion of the egg from the ovary, and the beginning of the *luteal phase* of the cycle. Once ovulation has occurred, fifteen days before the start of the next period, LH levels drop rapidly.

While FSH is around for the better part of the cycle, stimulating the production of estrogen and its attendant effects, LH comes out for just a short time, in spurts or pulses. LH production is turned off by the increasing levels of progesterone.

For the last two weeks of the cycle, estrogen and progesterone production are in balance to prepare the body for pregnancy.

Progesterone is made by the *corpus luteum,* the name given to the follicle once the egg has been expelled from the ovary. The corpus luteum then becomes an independent organ responsible for further support and preparation of the egg for fertilization. The progesterone made by the corpus luteum prevents other eggs from maturing, and keeps the uterine lining ready for implantation. More than 90 percent of the body's progesterone is made by this short-lived organ. If you get pregnant, the corpus luteum thrives and makes literally gallons of progesterone to nurture and sustain the fetus during the pregnancy. If you don't get pregnant, the corpus luteum shrinks and dies. With its demise, progesterone production—and thus circulating progesterone levels—wanes. The cycle has ended; you get your period. The fall of estrogen and progesterone levels is sensed by the hypothalamus. This signals the start of a new cycle, and the hypothalamus heralds it by secreting GnRH.

The cycle repeats itself every month until you either get pregnant or stop ovulating.

ESTROGEN, PROGESTERONE, AND TESTOSTERONE

Today, in the arsenal of medical knowledge, there are many sex hormone precursors, multiple "almost sex" hormones, and lots of wannabe sex hormones. There are only three true end-organ sex hormones: estrogen, progesterone, and testosterone. Both men and women have all three. The difference between men and women lies in the varying concentrations of these hormones circulating in the bloodstream.

Estrogen and progesterone are the dominant hormones in women. The dominant hormone in men is testosterone. A significant shortcoming in our understanding of hormones is the belief that estrogen, progesterone, and testosterone act independently of one another. The truth is that unless we totally incorporate into our understanding the inseparability of the three sex hormones, we cannot solve the problems caused by imbalances in their levels.

Estrogen

In women estrogen is made in the ovaries, the follicle around the ovum, the adrenal glands, and the fat cells.

Estrogen is not just one molecule, but rather a group of molecules. The three main estrogen molecules are estriol, estradiol, and estrone.

- **Estradiol (E_2).** Estradiol *(es-TRA-di-ol)* is the most active form of estrogen made by our ovaries, adrenals, and fat cells as we get older. Estradiol directly affects the functions of most of our body's organs. Practically every cell in our body houses on its surface receptors for estradiol. This means that estradiol can directly attach to every cell in our body and influence its function. This is the way estradiol affects organ function directly.

- **Estriol (E_3).** Estriol *(ES-tree-ol)* is the weakest and least active form of estrogens. It is mainly made by the placenta. It attaches to cell receptors making up hair, nails, skin, and mucosal membranes. It affects primarily the vaginal walls and has little effect on the heart or bones. In nonpregnant women, some estriol is made in the liver in small doses.

- **Estrone (E_1).** Estrone *(esTRONE)* in women is made after menopause primarily in fat cells from testosterone derivatives (androstenedione—*an-dro-STENE-di-own*) and also in the ovaries. While most data on estrone have been obtained from animal studies, human studies have shown that overweight older women have high circulating levels of estrone. A European study revealed higher levels of circulating estrone in women with breast cancer.

When we refer to estrogen, we refer to its three components as one. At times, this attempt to simplify creates errors in separating the individual functions of its components.

Although their combined actions present as one in what we know as estrogen, its component molecules have different potencies. For now, just remember that when I'm speaking of estrogen, I'm referring to all three components (estriol, estrone, estradiol) as one, unless otherwise specified. When I address treatment with natural hormones, however, I'll be separating the three estrogen molecules.

With the progression of the aging process, the ovaries stop producing estrogen on a regular basis, and the main source for the production of estrogen becomes the adrenal glands. Unused testosterone is also transformed into needed estrogen, and even estrogen stored in fat cells is called to action. Estrogen and progesterone are designed to balance each other, to keep each other in check.

We cannot live in a healthy state without their balanced presence in our bodies. As we begin to examine their individual effects, keep in mind that at no time does estrogen or progesterone act independently, in our body.

Estrogen makes everything grow. The positive effects of its action are that it:

- Makes the lining of the uterus grow, to prepare for pregnancy.
- Helps the breast tissues grow, in preparation for making milk.
- Causes the ovum to mature inside the ovary, to prepare for ovulation.
- Supports the growth of the follicle where the egg matures.
- Promotes the growth of the fetus.
- Keeps the vagina, the vulva, and the cervix well developed and moisturized.

- Promotes growth of underarm and pubic hair, and pigmentation of the nipples.
- Stimulates body fat accumulation, to help the fetus grow.
- Prevents bone destruction by bone-destroying cells (osteoclasts).
- Protects the body from hypertension by relaxing the lining of blood vessels.
- Stimulates the production of lipoprotein lipase, an enzyme that breaks down fat. The result is low cholesterol levels and a healthy balance between good (HDL) cholesterol and bad (LDL) cholesterol.
- Lowers insulin levels.
- Induces relaxation of blood vessels in the circulation in general, and the heart in particular.

The negative effects of the growth induced by estrogen unopposed (acting alone), without the balancing effects of progesterone, are:

- Increased accumulation of body fat.
- Increased water and salt retention.
- Interference with normal insulin release and blood sugar control.
- Increased risk of overgrowth of endometrium (lining of the uterus).
- Increased risk of overgrowth of breast tissue.
- Increased risk of anxiety and irritability.
- Increased risk of headaches.
- Increased risk of gallbladder disease.
- Increased incidence of blood clot formation.

Progesterone

Progesterone is made primarily by the corpus luteum (the follicle transformed after ovulation), and is a precursor to most sex hormones. Progesterone comes into action in the middle of the normal menstruating woman's cycle.

Stimulated by the release of LH (luteinizing hormone) in the form of pulses by the pituitary gland, progesterone is absolutely crucial to the survival of the ovum once fertilized. When pregnancy occurs, progesterone production increases rapidly and is taken over by the placenta. If the woman does not get pregnant, the corpus luteum shrinks, progesterone production falters, and menstruation arrives.

Progesterone is the precursor, or parent, of estrogen in the ovaries. The adrenal glands and testes also manufacture it. Progesterone is the precursor of testosterone, all androgens, and other adrenal hormones, making it extremely important for reasons far beyond its sex hormone role.

Progesterone's functions on the estrogen-progesterone team are to:

- Prepare the endometrium for implantation of the fertilized ovum.
- Ensure survival of the fetus in the uterus.
- Prevent water retention.
- Help use fat for energy at the cellular level.
- Serve as a natural antidepressant.
- Create a calming effect on the body.
- Help restore regular sleep patterns.
- Help keep insulin release in check and maintain even blood sugar levels.
- Prevent overgrowth of the endometrium.

- Prevent breast tissue overgrowth.
- Maintain sex drive.
- Maintain normal blood-clotting parameters.
- Protect against fibrocystic breasts.

Progesterone's negatives are few and easily balanced by estrogen:

- A sedating effect.
- Increased spotting and changes in bleeding patterns.
- Bloating, when taken in large quantities.
- Gastrointestinal discomfort.
- Acne.
- Hyperpigmentation of facial skin when exposed to sunlight.

Testosterone

The classic male hormone, testosterone is the third of the sex hormone trio. Made primarily in the testes and adrenals in men, and the adrenals, ovaries, and corpus luteum in women, testosterone is part of a class of hormones called *androgens*. These hormones have primarily masculinizing effects. Like estrogens, when we speak of androgens *(AN-dro-gens)*, we include more than one hormone: testosterone *(tes-TOS-te-rone)*, androstenediol *(an-dro-STENE-di-ol)*, dihydrotestosterone *(DI-hy-dro-tes-TOS-te-rone)*, andro-stanediol *(an-dro-STANE-di-ol)*, androstenedione *(an-dro-STENE-di-own)*, and dihydroepiandrosterone (DHEA) *(di-HY-dro-ep-i-an-dro-STER-one)*.

The most important role of testosterone is to provide male characteristics. Although this may appear straightforward, testosterone functions are of significance to women as well. Testosterone helps to:

- Promote muscle strength and exercise endurance.
- Improve libido.
- Increase energy levels.
- Improve sense of well-being.
- Increase body hair production.
- Produce enlargement of the penis and testes as well as clitoris.
- Improve sexual desire and fantasy.
- Improve bone density.

The negative effects of testosterone are due to overproduction or intake through either testosterone supplementation in pharmaceutical formulations or unsupervised androgen consumption. The side effects are similar to those of estrogen dominance, since testosterone transforms into estrogen when it's overabundant. These side effects include:

- Male pattern baldness.
- Increased facial hair.
- More aggressive behavior.
- Higher cholesterol levels.
- Too much clitoral enlargement.
- Involution of testes and penis.
- Growth of breast tissue in men.

We are only now starting to appreciate the importance of testosterone in men and women. While the balance of estrogen and progesterone is highly dependent on a cycle, we don't yet know how the balance of testosterone fits. As the story of hormones unfolds, I'm sure much more will come to light about testosterone.

Here, then, is the skeleton of hormone information I'll be building on.

Hormones are intimately involved in every body function. The amounts of hormones secreted are controlled by two glands in the brain—the hypothalamus and the pituitary. Hormones are produced by the sex organs: the ovaries, testes, and adrenal glands. There are three sex hormones: estrogen, progesterone, and testosterone. Their actions are interconnected and are both positive and negative. The balance and interaction among the sex hormones determine the presence or absence of symptoms.

In the chapters that follow, I promise you insights that can change your life for the better.

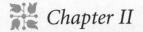 *Chapter II*

The Theory of Hormones

THE PHYSICAL DIFFERENCES

Now that we've looked at why, where, and how hormones are secreted, what regulates their production, and their relation to one another, let's move on to how they affect our lives.

Physical differences between males and females appear early in the development of the fetus in the uterus. As the fertilized egg is implanted into the soft, warm lining of the uterus, hormone levels skyrocket. By the time the first ultrasound is usually taken of the womb, around sixteen to twenty weeks, the sexual differences are already visible. High levels of hormones are mandatory for the survival and growth of the fetus. But once the baby is born, sexual differentiation comes to a screeching halt. For the following ten or twelve years, the difference between boys and girls is purely cultural and sociologic. Breasts don't grow, penises don't enlarge—physically, children are sexually indistinguishable.

What's going on here?

The marvelous sex hormones have decided to take a break. They've gone into a dormant phase while the baby grows from a newborn, to a toddler, to a young child. Other hormones have sent messages to the body to focus on other things. Growth of body organs, rapid increase in body size, development of the brain, and muscle coordination take precedence over the further development of sexual characteristics. This refocus is actually a blessing in disguise. Consider the confusion early puberty creates in our young girls. Recent research has been grappling with the increasing occurrence of early sexual development in seven- to ten-year-old girls—not easy to understand or deal with. Not only is this development worrisome from a physiologic standpoint, but it's concerning psychologically as well. We desperately need the dormancy period to develop. There's a good reason for the lag time: Anatomic and emotional maturation are critical and need time.

At puberty—for most, this occurs between the ages of eleven and thirteen—the sleepy sex hormones suddenly wake up. The sex glands—testes, ovaries, and adrenals—start making up for lost time and manufacture copious amounts of hormones. Our bodies become awash with sex hormones. Estrogen, progesterone, and testosterone are flooding the system. The rapid transformation from girl into woman, and from boy into man, has begun with a vengeance.

From Girl to Woman, from Boy to Man

If our genetic makeup is within normal limits (as is true in most people), these increasing levels of well-balanced estrogen, progesterone, and testosterone translate into the emergence of a young adult. In medical terms, this change is referred to as the appearance of secondary sexual characteristics.

During middle school, when your children are undergoing maturity physicals, the doctor looks for the appearance of these secondary sexual characteristics to determine what is considered normal development. While to the naked eye we see growing breasts, pubic and armpit hair, and adult-smelling perspiration, few of us consciously realize that it's our sex hormones working on the inside that are creating these changes.

Inside our bodies, when a critical balance of estrogen and progesterone has been reached, voilà, the girl starts to ovulate (release an egg). Every month, she gets her period, and is now physically ready to have children of her own.

Boys follow the same path. Who hasn't heard the cracking voice of the twelve-year-old turn from a soprano to a frog overnight? And how remarkable it is to watch the appearance of facial hair and the growth spurt that turns your little boy into a towering man. What we don't see so readily is how hormones have also brought on the growth of pubic hair and enlargement of the penis and testes.

And these changes address only the impact hormones have on the physical development of the boy and girl. Many emotional changes are also directly correlated to changes in hormones. Studies have shown that although environment has a significant impact on emotional outlook, it's hormones that turn women into nesters, desirous of having babies, while men continue their focus on sports and competitive endeavors. Children who suffer from hormone deficiency syndromes maintain a neutral emotional attitude in life. They don't exhibit either male- or female-specific emotional traits. Remember the androgynous Pat from *Saturday Night Live*? A perfect example of a human being not under the influence of hormones.

HOW HORMONES KEEP HUMANS FROM BECOMING AN ENDANGERED SPECIES

During the first eight to ten years of life, our sex hormones are in hibernation because they're preparing for the first big bang—adolescence.

Teenagers

The term *adolescence* doesn't explain why the sweet ten-year-old who yesterday held your hand and said, "I love you, Mommy," suddenly woke up at the age of twelve convinced that you're a moron and an embarrassment. The term *adolescence* just gives us a name for this inexplicable behavior. There is a critical but physiological reason for the irrationality of adolescent behavior—the "hormone storm."

For years, parents have justified their teenage son's or daughter's behavior with the catchphrase, "It's the hormones." Well, that certainly is the truth. The only problem is that when we refer to this hormone storm, we think in terms of their behavior on the outside and their overflowing sexuality. We readily attribute to hormones teenagers' pimples and their short fuses when it comes to parental advice, but we fail to realize another much bigger effect hormones have on our teens.

We rarely notice how incredibly healthy they are. They recover from the flu in twenty-four hours; they can eat 5,000 calories of junk food a day and not gain an ounce. We're painfully aware that teens can sleep for twenty hours on Sunday after staying up all night on Friday and Saturday—then hardly sleep at all the rest of the week.

We just take that for granted. We say it's youth.

We watch in awe of their boundless energy, but we don't make the connection between this zest for life and their hormones. Yes, it is youth, but youth is due in large part to the overabundance of hormones in the body. Scientifically speaking, estrogen and testosterone rev up the system and stimulate energy production at the cellular level. The teen's metabolic rate is high; things are happening. Muscles are built overnight, and the aggressive and often optimistic outlook on life this imparts to young men and women makes them feel immortal. Progesterone balances the two energizing hormones by softening their impact, moderating the amount of growth and energy produced, and allowing for rest and renewal. This explosion of hormones occurs in the adolescent's body for one reason, and one reason only: to prepare for reproduction.

Don't get me wrong—I don't want to relegate human beings to being nothing more than baby machines. But that's precisely what hormones do and how our species survives. Our hormones don't care that we are evolved, intelligent humans. All they care about is that we perpetuate the species. What we have to understand is how our hormones work to protect us, and how to identify when and why they fall short of that protective goal. Then we can correct their mistakes with treatments that are safe and return us to a younger self.

Twenties

We're now into our late teens, early twenties. We're in better control of our hormones—not that we've mastered them; instead, they have mastered us. We have learned to live with our new identity. Socially, we can get along with adults better (although we still doubt their worth); we are integrating into society.

So what happens next?

We search for a mate, someone to have our children with. That's where being in an advanced society gives us the edge. We don't have to rely on just genetic makeup. Socially, we have fun, focus on our looks, get an education, find a great job, buy fancy clothes, join a health club and become buff. We do whatever it takes to become attractive to the opposite sex. There are cultural reasons why we do all this, but above it all, it's to fulfill our mission to reproduce.

On the outside, our social development defines our

behavior, while on the inside our hormones are protecting us from harm. *Heart attacks, cancer,* and *strokes* are not part of the twenty-year-old's vocabulary. If they occur, they're rare. This great health is due to the fact that our hormones are watching over us. They have created a protective bubble around us. They keep us immortal. We have a goal—the Perpetuation of the Human Species—to fulfill, and our hormones will make sure we achieve it.

This is the time in life when most women get pregnant. This event reveals a clear picture of how hormones operate. When we're pregnant, we are protected from harm: Our estrogen and progesterone levels are sky-high. We don't get sick, we just glow. We gain weight but have no problems as a result. Our bones get stronger, our hair gets thicker, our skin is wrinkle-free, and all because our increased levels of hormones are protecting us.

High estrogen stimulates bone production, synchronizes heart function, washes away cholesterol deposits from our arteries, and stimulates serotonin production in our brains, which keeps our spirits high. High testosterone stimulates muscle cell growth, protects our heart cells from toxic damage, and maintains our metabolic rate at a high level so we don't get fat or sluggish. During pregnancy, hormone levels are astronomic—and it's exactly during this time that we are healthy and thriving.

Despite the findings of some studies, the question remains: If estrogen were to cause cancer, wouldn't the incidence of cancer skyrocket during pregnancy? This is a time in our lives when we're actually living a scientific experiment—we're watching how high estrogen and progesterone levels affect our lives. If we stay healthy during pregnancy, we have proven that estrogen made by our bodies is not a dangerous hormone but rather a safe protector of our youth and health. Statistically speaking, pregnant women don't usually get cancer or have heart attacks, and they have thick bones and skin that's wrinkle-free.

Thirties

We've found a mate, started a family, and hormonally speaking are on automatic pilot for the next fifteen-plus years. Some of us have no children, others have one or more, and our hormones follow the changes set by the presence or absence of pregnancy. While we're busy raising a family, Mother Nature wants our species to thrive and survive. This simple fact translates into a fairly constant hormone balance with rare glitches in the system. Our periods are fairly regular, we maintain our weight, we sleep well and look young and are still full of energy. Because it takes our offspring a minimum of fifteen years to become self-sustaining, our hormone balance and the state of our health have to parallel this timeline. Scientifically, hormones will continue protecting us for the fifteen years we need to raise our children. Emotionally and economically, our society has extended the time our children need our support. But even from that standpoint, eventually our children become self-sufficient. They do grow up. By the time they're off to college, starting their own search for a mate, or beginning a career, they leave behind not only an empty nest but also a hormonally drained parent, who's now forty to fifty years old.

Forties and Fifties

How often do you hear about the couple looking forward to shipping the last kid off to college, making plans for early retirement to Florida to play golf—and then, bang! The wife gets breast cancer. Or, bang! The husband has a heart attack.

Fortunately, for most the transition is not so traumatic.

Not everyone has a heart attack or gets cancer when they're ready to retire. Still, lots of changes occur at this point in your life that must be addressed. There you are, ready to exhale, to reclaim or maybe start a new life. Instead, you start sweating in the middle of the night and find that you can no longer deal with the simplest of problems. Overnight, you become a human blimp, your sex drive is gone, and your bones ache so much, you'd just as soon stay in bed and pull the covers over your head.

What's going on here? It's a dirty trick Mother Nature has just played on us. Our job is done; we have accomplished our goal. We reproduced ourselves, we ensured the propagation of our species. So Mother Nature will now proceed to get rid of us. She ruthlessly removes the high-octane fuel—our hormones—that protected us from harm and kept us healthy when we were "useful." Removal of the hormones results in one main thing: aging.

When we age, we have heart problems, get cancer, have strokes, are beset with chronic illnesses, and are stooped over with thinning brittle bones, failing eyesight, and waning memory. So what's the main difference between those who are youthful and those who are aging? That's right, you have it—it's hormones. If you're youthful (and useful, according to Mother Nature), here is your profile: You're brimming with hormones, you're pimply, you're menstruating, you're moody, your perspiration has a strong and pungent odor, and you want to have sex—all the time. This picture might be simplistic, but I assure you, it's also a sure way to identify your position on the food chain.

Once you've had kids and they're grown, you're no longer useful, and your hormones depart. The dwindling hormone levels cause you to get depressed and bloated. Sex becomes a chore, and your skin starts to sag. Even plastic surgery can't hide that shar-pei look. Then poof, one day you're gone.

As long as you're young and have the potential to have babies, estrogen, progesterone, and testosterone will protect you. Ovaries, testes, and adrenals will produce large quantities of hormones. When you're done having babies, and they've grown up and can physically take care of themselves, you're no longer needed. So hormone production just turns off.

Your body will betray you, and you will get old.

It sounds pretty depressing.

But never fear—all of that is just theoretical physiology, and it doesn't have to apply to our generation any longer. After all, we can put a man on the moon and connect the world via the Internet. Certainly, we can fool Mother Nature and extend our existence by replenishing our hormones into old age. We can delay our aging process; we don't have to feel horrible just because we're getting older. If we just supplement our hormones, we can prevent our decline for a long time. We simply have to be careful with the kind of hormones we use.

Synthetic replacements, in my opinion, aren't as effective as natural hormones. I have treated many patients who, with the help of natural hormones, are defying age, feeling and looking young at sixty, seventy, even eighty. You too can be one of these fortunate people.

Just keep reading.

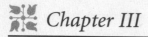

Chapter III

The Symptoms of Hormone Imbalance Occur at All Ages

Chapter 2 contained an important lesson: During our reproductive years, we're usually pretty healthy. We stay healthy mainly because the high levels of sex hormones we produce protect us from illness.

Of course, even though most young people are healthy (statistically speaking) and wellness is the rule, the system isn't perfect. Identifying the imperfections in our hormone balance that occur during our youth opens the door for us to protect ourselves from rapid aging as we get older.

Hormones do not protect us from *all* harm. Like a computer system, the human body does crash on occasion. The hormone balance gets thrown off even in the healthiest of people at the peak of their youth. When the hormone balance is off, we often experience symptoms. Not every young woman will experience symptoms of hormone imbalance, but many women will at different times in their lives. Our ability to manage our own menopause, with its significant hormone deficiencies, requires an understanding of the concept that episodes of hormone imbalance occur regardless of age.

When our hormones are in balance, our bodies, for the most part, function like well-oiled engines, but when the balance is off we become squeaky wheels. Minute changes in hormone levels—almost imperceptible to even the most sensitive of lab tests—create significant symptoms. It's the suddenness of change in the levels of hormones that gives us symptoms at all stages and ages in life.

Laboratory tests cannot measure these infinitesimal fluctuations. They offer little help as we desperately try to right our lives while being carried along on the roller-coaster ride of our hormones. If no diagnosable disease exists, conventional medicine cannot treat us.

Despite high-tech tests and scientific breakthroughs, the best diagnostic tool in life remains "how you feel." Let's use how you feel as a guide to identify the symptoms, and then let's connect the symptoms to the particular hormone imbalances that cause them. A careful examination of the symptoms of hormone imbalance as they appear throughout your life reveals more than you think. Notice how the same symptoms you experienced at twenty—and ignored—become overwhelming at forty, and then deadly at sixty.

It's crucial to connect the similarity in symptoms at all ages with hormone imbalance. If we connect them, we can treat them. If we treat them effectively—meaning *with natural hormones*—we can help prevent aging and disease.

Identified by decades, symptoms of hormone imbalance become easier to understand and quicker to treat.

SYMPTOMS OF HORMONE IMBALANCE IN THE TEENS

Acne
Mood swings

Acne

Michelle is fourteen. Her mother brought her to see me because she has acne. She had started her periods the year before—a little late, according to her mother, as her friends had started between eleven and twelve. Before Michelle had her period, her skin was as smooth and clear as a porcelain doll's. When her period started, it was like something wreaked havoc on her face. She woke up one morning with her face covered with pimples. Not just pimples, but large, swollen, painful, and unsightly bumps littering her chin, her forehead, and even her back. Michelle was devastated. She didn't want to leave the house and became depressed.

Acne Is a Symptom of Hormone Imbalance

Hormones hit their stride with the beginning of menstruation. Whether the girl is eleven or seventeen, when she starts menstruating, her ovaries release an egg every month, and her estrogen and progesterone levels follow a cycle. (See chapter 1.)

Occasionally, though, something goes awry. It takes time for the body to adjust to being on a cycle. During this adjustment period, the balance of estrogen, progesterone, and testosterone isn't always finely tuned. This imbalance—the highs and lows of rapid changes in hormone levels—sometimes presents itself clinically as acne. High levels of estrogen and testosterone create a perfect environment for this bane of teens. Both estrogen and testosterone make oil glands grow, and the increase in progesterone after ovulation offers a fertile ground for pimple growth.

Although not a life-threatening situation, acne is unsightly and makes young girls and boys, who are already undergoing identity problems, uncomfortable.

Mood Swings

A straight-A student, Louise was the pride and joy of her parents. Beautiful, bright, and friendly, she seemed to be sailing through the tough teen years while others were struggling. Her mother, a longtime patient of mine, often told me how lucky she felt to have a child like Louise. She was an example for her younger siblings.

Things continued well until Louise turned seventeen. It was "extremely sudden," her mother told me when she came to my office, desperate for advice. Louise's personality had dramatically changed. What once was an environment of happy, open communication turned into door slamming and isolation. A different Louise emerged.

While still a good student, Louise stopped talking to her parents, her siblings, and most of her friends. She became morose and grim. Her clothes were dark and dreary. She sported purple hair. She spent hours in her room, on the phone, blasting the stereo and the TV, and often did not come down for dinner. When asked what was wrong, Louise went on the attack. Everything wrong in her life was her parents' fault. Louise's mother took her to a therapist for five sessions. Louise spent the time blankly staring at the wall or at her green fingernails.

Mood Swings Are Caused by Hormone Imbalance

All too often, hormone imbalance during the teen years is misinterpreted, incorrectly treated, or just plain ignored. All it takes is a sudden change in the balance of the levels of estrogen and progesterone, and poof!—you have emotional problems. An imbalance of progesterone in the second half of the month, after ovulation, may bring about depression in your otherwise pleasant teen. If estrogen and testosterone are overabundant, the result is a very aggressive, contrary, adversarial teen.

It's the fluctuation—the sudden surges followed by precipitous drops in hormones—that cause the otherwise docile teen to change moods with the speed of light, or the clear-skinned youth to sprout a crop of pimples the day of the prom.

Stress Makes Hormone Balance Change

Yes, it may be stress that makes the pimples grow, and stress certainly can change people's personalities. Stress causes immediate and drastic changes in hormone levels. The best-known reaction for dealing with stress is the "fight or flight" mechanism. Our ancestors who lived in caves and had to protect themselves from attack by wild animals and other dangers reacted instinctually through their hormones. They didn't have the ability or wherewithal to think before they acted. At the core of the mechanism that saved their lives was a simple but most powerful hormone.

Cortisol is the hormone our adrenal glands make to protect us from danger. It's released every time our body or mind thinks we're about to get hurt. To the body, stress means danger. When cortisol is released to help us run away from harm, our immune system is activated. Progesterone levels drop, and insulin levels rise. This is important, because the more time we spend in our lives under stress, the more out of balance our hormones become. The results are increased energy production, accumulation of toxic waste products, faster aging, and ultimately permanent organ damage as manifested in the form of chronic diseases.

Our hormones prepare us to fight or run away from danger when we're under major stress. This mechanism works well in the wild, or in situations where stress is a matter of life and death. It doesn't work as well in a world where stress is about who's more popular in school. The cortisol release in response to the "fight or flight" perception of stress, no longer appropriate in our society, creates hormone imbalances that show up as acne and mood swings when we're young. The teen's body will try to right this hormone imbalance. But the symptoms appear so quickly that it may take months or years to get the overall balance back in check.

During this time, parents desperately seek help. The help need not come from antidepressants or other heavy-duty synthetic medications. Learning to cope with stress and eliminating the spikes of cortisol levels are the first steps. Understanding the teen's reaction to stress means understanding this old, outdated, but seriously destructive mechanism, and protecting the child from its untoward effects. Supplementation with natural hormones is the next step. Natural hormones (bioidentical) are so similar to the teen's own hormones, and their action is so gentle, that they can help right the balance and eliminate the symptoms. Finally, re-creating the ideal hormone balance helps naturally eliminate the symptoms and boosts the teen's spirits while his or her own hormone manufacturing system rights itself.

SYMPTOMS OF HORMONE IMBALANCE IN THE TWENTIES

Postpartum depression
Night sweats
Infertility

Postpartum Depression

Our twenties are a joyous time. Beautifully synchro-nized, our hormones keep us vibrant, healthy, and ready to reproduce. And that we do. In our twenties, most of us start our families and have children. But while we usually sail through childbirth and its aftermath without a hitch, occasional problems arise. When they do, we're left baffled and without answers or—worse yet—with the wrong answers.

Here's the story of a patient who exemplifies what too many women go through at a time when joy should prevail.

Marcia was twenty-five and had just embarked on a career in advertising. She had been my patient since her early teens and had never had medical or psychological problems. She got married at twenty-three to her college sweetheart, who was on the corporate fast track. After a happy year together, they decided to start a family. Marcia's mother was available to care for the baby, hence they had no worries about conflict between career and family.

Marcia gave birth to a healthy baby boy. Within a month, though, she started showing signs of clinical depression. Everything was fine on the outside—the baby, the marriage; even Marcia's body was quickly returning to prepregnancy shape. But Marcia was not completely back to her normal self. She had no interest in sex, no interest in returning to her job; she was short tempered and impatient with the baby. She found herself crying at the drop of a hat. One day, she started having terrible thoughts, thoughts of death. She was afraid she had cancer or another deadly disease. She feared she would not live to see her baby grow up. These thoughts wouldn't leave. She couldn't sleep; she repeatedly woke up at 5 A.M., her heart pounding and her stomach tied in knots. She went to a psychiatrist and was correctly diagnosed with postpartum depression.

Night Sweats

When I had my first baby, I was twenty-seven years old. I was healthy and had a great pregnancy. One night when my little girl was six weeks old, I was awakened not by the usual crying of the baby, but by an incredible night sweat. I thought the worst. I thought I was dying of tuberculosis or a major blood infection. By morning, I was feeling better and, having no fever or other signs of illness, I promptly forgot about the incident. When I returned to work a few weeks later, I remembered what had happened and started asking my fellow doctors if they had heard about similar episodes. No one had. I looked it up in the medical literature and found no mention of it.

As the years passed and I became a specialist in hormones, I realized that the night sweat episode I experienced was not unusual and was a result of the sudden drop in hormone levels that follow the delivery of a baby. As I developed clinical methods for treatments of hormone imbalances, I thought about this episode. Routinely, I started to ask my young patients about episodes of night sweats after having babies. More than 60 percent of those questioned answered yes.

Sudden Changes in Hormone Balance Cause Symptoms

All these stories are about symptoms of hormone imbalance. Whether it's postpartum depression or night sweats in a young woman, the cause is almost always the same—a sudden change in hormone balance.

The high levels of estrogen and progesterone our healthy bodies make to support the growth and development of the fetus in the womb suddenly drop when the baby is born, and the extra hormones are no longer needed. This sudden drop in hormone levels, albeit normal, can manifest as depression or night sweats in some women.

Every woman who has a baby experiences a sudden drop in hormone levels. When these levels drop, some women respond with symptoms, while others don't. It isn't a matter of normal or abnormal, it just is. In fact, the drop in hormone levels after childbirth protects women from far greater harm. What would happen if, once the baby was born, the sky-high levels of estrogen and progesterone didn't budge? Remember, the hormone levels are high in order to maintain and support the growth of the fetus in the womb. Once the baby is born, we must get rid of the extra hormones as quickly as possible. Otherwise, they'd kill us. High estrogen would make every cell continue its growth. The constant stimulation by the hormones of pregnancy would undoubtedly end our lives on short notice.

Placed in proper perspective, then, depression or night sweats is a small price to pay to rid the body of hormones that can become deadly after the end of pregnancy. Still, sometimes the body overshoots the balance. If there's too much of a drop, too suddenly, in a sensitized or genetically predisposed woman, symptoms will swamp her.

I'm not trying to make light of postpartum depression or night sweats. They are real and they create an enormous amount of discomfort. I only want to establish the all-important connection between the fluctuation in levels of hormones and symptoms.

Infertility

Maureen is a successful thirty-six-year-old banker. She got pregnant without difficulty with her first child. About three years ago, Maureen and her husband decided that their healthy six-year-old son needed a sibling. Because their first experience with conception was such a piece of cake, by the time

Maureen realized she wasn't getting pregnant, a year had passed. With her type A personality, she went into panic mode. She immediately made an appointment with a renowned infertility specialist and underwent a comprehensive battery of tests. Everything was anatomically normal with her and with her husband—and yet she wasn't pregnant. She finally conceived two years later, when a fertility specialist placed her on natural progesterone for two months after ovulation occurred.

Infertility is an enormous concern in the field of obstetrics and gynecology. Many causes for infertility have been identified. And it should come as no surprise that many are connected to hormone imbalance. Examples include:

- Inadequate progesterone production by the corpus luteum.

- Imbalance between levels of estrogen and progesterone, making the implantation of the ovum into the uterus impossible.

- Hormone imbalance that makes the egg unfriendly toward the sperm, not allowing penetration and thus preventing fertilization.

Hormone problems can be at the root of infertility not only in women in their thirties and beyond, but in twenty-year-olds as well.

SYMPTOMS OF HORMONE IMBALANCE IN THE THIRTIES

Bloating
PMS
Migraines
Breast tenderness
Decreasing attention span
Weight gain

Let's move on to our thirties. Notice the increasing number of symptoms lining up under the above heading? To better understand what happens to our body in our thirties, we must revisit the function of the corpus luteum we addressed in chapter 1, and the changes that occur as we get older.

Remember, the corpus luteum exists to manufacture progesterone and get the body ready for pregnancy. If we don't get pregnant, the production of estrogen and progesterone shuts down. The corpus luteum dies, and we get our period.

The same scenario goes on every month for more than thirty years. Thus, if you looked at a woman in her thirties from the standpoint of the regularity of her menstrual cycle, she usually looks the same as a woman in her twenties. But that's where the similarities end. (Apologies to all those thirty-year-olds who physically look twenty.)

For the moment, I'm looking at pure physiology. Both outside and in, a woman in her thirties doesn't look as youthful as a woman in her twenties. While a few crow's-feet may begin to appear around her eyes, and her hips may be a little wider, more significant signs of aging appear inside her body.

The corpus luteum does not manufacture progesterone as high in quality as it did in the twenties. This is crucial.

The decrease in the quality of progesterone translates into the increasing appearance of symptoms of hormone imbalance in the thirties. Let's take Olga, for example.

Olga is a thirty-five-year-old I've been seeing since I started working with hormones. She has three children—ages twelve, eight, and six. A single mother, she works as a substitute teacher in the Bronx. At night and on the weekends, Olga used to be a cocktail waitress to supplement her income. When she first came to see me, she was very upset. She had gained twenty-five pounds since the birth of her last child, now six, and couldn't lose it no matter what she did. Her waitressing days were over. She'd gone from a size 6 to a size 14. She exercised, assured me she ate sensibly (vegetables, fruit, protein, and very little pasta, rice, potatoes, or bread)—but nothing happened.

The more obsessed she became with her diet, the more she seemed unable to lose a pound. And adding insult to injury, in the last six months Olga had developed the most incredible food cravings. She never used to like sweets. Now she could kill for a piece of chocolate; she had a hiding place in her kitchen where she kept a stash that even her kids didn't know about.

Before her periods, Olga got migraines, her breasts swelled into painful balloons, and she became a "raving lunatic" (her words). In the past, Olga said, she was a patient woman, and her kids could do no wrong in her eyes. They're good kids, she assured me. Now, however, if her oldest entered the house with dirty boots and failed to wipe his feet, she flew into a rage. If the same thing happened during the first or second week of her cycle, Olga told me, she was a different person. During that point in the cycle, she was conscious of her rage and could control it. However, as her period neared, she lost the ability to control her temper.

Olga is—like most women in their thirties—starting to experience hormone imbalance episodes that are more frequent, consistent, and intense than those she had in her twenties.

Bloating

Bloating is a symptom that occurs a few days before the start of menstruation and disappears around the fourth day of the cycle. It's characterized by swelling in the midsection of the body and extremities. Common complaints include tight-feeling pants, abdominal discomfort after even a small meal, tight rings, dents left on the shins by snug-fitting socks, swollen eyes in the morning, and ballooning midriff soon after eating salty foods.

Unnecessary water retention in our tissues is what causes us to bloat. Water retention is triggered by increased levels of estrogen unbalanced by progesterone. Elevated levels of estrogen increase water retention in the individual cells, and—whether they're in your intestines, in your stomach, or the fat cells on your belly—the result is bloating.

PMS

How about PMS? What about premenstrual dysphoric disorder—PMDD? We hear more about these every day; are we in the throes of an epidemic of psychiatric illness?

As women enter their thirties, the range of incapacitating syndromes surrounding menstrual cycles grows. For years, I wondered why. I thought it might be because women become more aware of their bodies in their thirties. Then I looked specifically at women in their teens and twenties. When I asked, patients invariably admitted to suffering from the same symptoms, only to lesser degrees.

I began reading every piece of conventional medical and consumer literature on the topic of PMS and PMDD. It seems you can find an article to agree or disagree with every theory put forth.

So what's the answer? What causes PMDD and PMS?

You might have guessed. Hormone imbalance. This time the culprit is lack of progesterone. In chapter 1, we learned that the corpus luteum makes progesterone. This continues as we age, but the progesterone becomes much poorer in quality. If there isn't enough high-quality progesterone circulating in the bloodstream, the estrogen (also on the decline, but not as much yet) is free to wreak havoc. Put another way, high levels of estrogen unbalanced by progesterone manifests as PMS and PMDD.

No, you're not losing your mind; you're just losing your much-needed progesterone. When you don't have enough progesterone circulating, estrogen is the dominant hormone. Estrogen in overabundance makes you angry, edgy, short tempered, and anxious. At the same time, estrogen increases the water content of the cells in your brain, making you groggy, fuzzy, and unfocused.

In summary, too much estrogen is the culprit for PMS and associated so-called dysphoric disorders.

Breast Tenderness

Low progesterone and high, unopposed estrogen right before your period causes tender, sore breasts. Estrogen holds on to water in the cells and makes the breast tissue grow. When progesterone is not there to balance the estrogen, you can get sore, swollen breasts before your periods. Notorious for this situation are the anovulatory cycles of aging women. During months when you don't ovulate any longer, progesterone production diminishes rapidly after the middle of the cycle. Since no egg matures, no corpus luteum develops, hence no progesterone. These are the months in which you may experience severe swollen, tender breasts, PMS, and bloating.

Migraines

Fluctuation in hormone levels produce changes in the walls of blood vessels. Such changes can also affect the vessels of the scalp—they widen, and we experience headaches. Estrogen induces dilation of the blood vessels everywhere in the body, including the scalp. Progesterone balances it. When estrogen is left unopposed, the blood vessels stay widened, leading to headaches.

Women with a genetic predisposition to migraines usually start experiencing severe headaches around the time they start menstruating. As they get older, these women experience more headaches—which often become more incapacitating. Again, this is because progesterone is not being made, either because ovulation has ceased, or because the corpus luteum in older women does not make good-quality progesterone.

Often, women on birth control pills or synthetic hormone replacement complain of severe migraines. Birth control pills are made with synthetic estrogens and synthetic progestins. They work by preventing ovulation from occurring. They accomplish this by keeping estrogen levels high enough that the ovum does not mature. It's an override mechanism. The trade-off is high estrogen levels, combining the estrogen the body manufactures with synthetic estrogens. Remember the effect of estrogen on the blood vessels? Widening, dilation of these vessels, translates into severe migraines that often limit the use of birth control pills.

Decreasing Attention Span

How often do you walk into a room and wonder why you went there to begin with? How often do you sit in a meeting listening intently to the speaker, only to realize that you just lost the point of the talk? How often do you start a project and give up too soon? How come this doesn't happen routinely to a twenty-year-old? These are questions many of my patients in their thirties ask. Are they experiencing the first signs of Alzheimer's? Are these "senior moments"?

Twenty-five years of clinical experience and the supporting scientific literature offer simple, commonsense answers: You have more information and responsibility, more stress and fewer outlets, less time to fit in all your life's activities, and decreasing estrogen and progesterone levels. All these factors produce a constellation of symptoms that can add up to decreasing attention span. They are often correctable. Taking medications, or worrying about aging and the potential for chronic disability, just aren't necessary for the average healthy thirty-year-old whose life is too busy and whose hormones need a bit of help.

Weight Gain

As I'm sure you're aware, many women in their thirties gain weight. All too often, these women can no longer maintain their ideal weight. When asked, they often identify the time they lost the battle of the bulge as the birth of their last child. After the last child is born, many women become unable to lose those extra 20 or 30 pounds.

Bad diet? Lack of exercise? No sleep?

Yes, probably.

But the biggest culprit is often hormone imbalance. Those beautifully fine-tuned hormones are now starting to go on the blink.

Food cravings that never occurred before are all too common in our thirties. I see women who tell me, "I never used to like sweets, but now it's all about the dessert menu." There is a very significant connection between our estrogen and progesterone levels and insulin. The first time I spoke of insulin was a few pages back, when I addressed stress in teens. There I noted that cortisol, the fight or flight hormone, stimulates insulin release. For the teen, this is a small problem; as we get older, it becomes a much bigger issue.

Insulin is the hormone (yes, it is a hormone) made in the pancreas. This little-known long, thin organ is neatly tucked away under the left side of our rib cage, and controls blood sugar levels. When insulin is released into our bloodstream, the blood sugar level drops instantly. If too much insulin is released, the blood sugar level overshoots and drops too low. This sudden drop in blood sugar leaves us weak, woozy, shaky on the inside, sweaty on the outside, and craving sweets. Only maintaining balanced levels of sugar in our bloodstream can stop insulin from being released by the pancreas. So if we eat a candy bar that is all processed sugar, it gets easily absorbed into our bloodstream, and the sugar level shoots up—rapidly, causing insulin levels to go up as well. If instead we eat protein or fiber, it takes longer for the blood sugar level to go up, so the insulin level doesn't spike.

The constant fluctuation of insulin in our bloodstream is deadly to our system. The more insulin, the more cortisol, the more wear and tear on the body, and the more quickly we age.

So what does all this have to do with our sex hormones? Insulin release is dependent upon sugar—but also on progesterone and estrogen blood levels. Estrogen stimulates insulin release; progesterone tempers it.

As the quality of progesterone made by the corpus luteum becomes poorer, circulating estrogen is not balanced by progesterone, more insulin is released more rapidly and more often, and the craving for sugar often becomes more and more uncontrollable regardless of your body's requirements.

Did you ever notice around your period how desperately you need to eat every three hours? It's because the estrogen unbalanced by the disappearing progesterone precipitates insulin release and a sudden drop in sugar levels. Unfortunately, this is a cascade effect leading to aging.

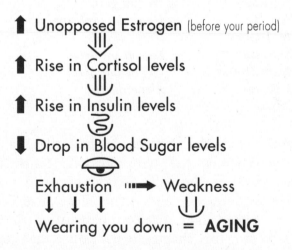

↑ Unopposed Estrogen (before your period)

↑ Rise in Cortisol levels

↑ Rise in Insulin levels

↓ Drop in Blood Sugar levels

Exhaustion ⟶ Weakness

↓ ↓ ↓

Wearing you down = **AGING**

It's a known fact that women tolerate low sugar levels much better than men. While men need sugar levels around 100, women feel normal with blood sugar levels around 60. This accounts for the very delicate sugar balance in women and its wide range of normalcy. When the hormone balance is off, insulin responds by spiking out of control. This situation causes sugar levels to plummet, and women quickly become hypoglycemic—feeling weak and sweaty and, above all, craving sugars.

The older the woman, the less finely tuned the hormone balance, the more symptoms start to appear, and the more rapidly the aging process advances.

SYMPTOMS AND DISEASES ASSOCIATED WITH HORMONE IMBALANCE IN THE FORTIES AND BEYOND

Acne	*Mood swings*
Sleep disorders	*Bloating*
Migraines	*Weight gain*
Hair loss	*Digestive problems*
Hot flashes	*Night sweats*
Depression	*Loss of sex drive*
Heart disease	*High cholesterol*
Bone loss	*Alzheimer's*
Cancer	

Let's continue into the next decade, the forties. By now, it should be obvious that symptoms associated with menopause occur throughout life. Only at menopause when they increase in frequency and occur all at once do we become overwhelmed and notice their destructive effects. If you look back over this chapter, you'll notice that almost every symptom under the "Forties and Beyond" heading has appeared before. It's a bit reassuring to see that these are not sudden developments; we experience all of them at other times in our lives.

Mary is forty, successful in business, and happily married. Her health history is impeccable. She has never missed a day of work, nor has she been absent from the gym more than one week at a time. Lately, though, Mary has been experiencing strange symptoms. She gets an occasional hot flash, especially the day before her period starts. Sometimes she wakes up in the middle of the night and has a night sweat, or just has to urinate very badly. She never liked sweets, and yet over the past few months she's been developing a sweet tooth. When she went to see her doctor for her annual physical and told her about these symptoms, the doctor just shrugged them off. She's too young and her periods are regular—no reason for concern. Everything is okay . . . or is it?

Actually it isn't. What Mary is experiencing is all too common in her age group. As we enter our late thirties and early forties, the amount and quality of progesterone made by the corpus luteum decrease, and symptoms develop. It doesn't mean we are menopausal; it just means we may need a little more progesterone to balance our hormones.

Sonia is forty-seven. She has three grown children. She's happily married to her high school sweetheart, and they have a good life together. Unfortunately for Sonia, her genetics are against her. Her mother died at forty-three from a heart attack; an older sister, now fifty-four, had breast cancer; and her fifty-eight-year-old brother has Alzheimer's, a heavy load to carry. Yet Sonia has been taking all the necessary precautions to soften the impact of her genetic makeup. She eats a well-balanced diet, exercises regularly, and goes to yoga class once a week.

She keeps up with medical advances in prevention. She had a bone density test at forty-five. She gets yearly mammograms, cholesterol measurements, and Pap smears. Because she was doing everything right, she hoped life would stay on track for her. And so it did, until she started having hot flashes ten and twenty times a day, became depressed, and lost her sex drive—all within the span of six months. When her periods started to change, Sonia took over-the-counter menopause treatments religiously. Within a short time, she was taking as many as thirty pills a day. Her doctor recommended birth control pills as hormone replacement therapy, but Sonia refused, as she was scared of the potential side effects. As the months progressed, Sonia found herself in a tailspin, trying to catch up with her constantly increasing number of symptoms and frustrated by the lack of solutions offered.

Sonia came to me looking for a solution to her hormone problems. We worked together to improve her chances of beating the odds against her genetic load. She went on the program in *The Hormone Solution*. Combining the beneficial results obtained through natural hormone supplementation, diet, exercise, and lifestyle, Sonia felt better and more confident of having taken a proactive role in her future.

Hot Flashes

Hot flashes are the bane of women in menopause. But women experience hot flashes during their twenties and thirties as well. Because their frequency increases at menopause, and that's when they get addressed.

Hot flashes are the immediate result of the blood vessel dilation that occurs when unopposed estrogen dominates the hormone picture. The pituitary gland then releases pulses of luteinizing hormone, hoping to push the ovaries to make more progesterone. The temperature-control mechanism in our body short-circuits because of the estrogen dominance, and we get hot.

Auras (premonitions) of hot flashes are common. Women report that almost every time they have a hot flash, they know it's coming. Also, some women experience extended flashes—a few minutes—while others describe only a few seconds. Still, nearly everyone agrees that hot flashes are horrible—and that we'll do almost anything to get rid of them.

Depression

The presence of normal levels of estrogen, well balanced by progesterone, stimulates the production and the release of serotonin, the ultimate feel-good hormone in the brain. The higher the serotonin levels, the happier we are. When we enter menopause, however, estrogen and progesterone levels drop, and serotonin follows. On the outside, the aging process is robbing us of youthful looks and we're starting to feel like rickety old chairs. Between the drop in estrogen and serotonin, the decreasing quality and quantity of progesterone we make on the inside, and the physical changes of aging on the outside, depression rears its ugly head more and more with advancing age.

Sleep Disorders

Decreasing levels of progesterone before our periods and as we age bring about all types of problems with sleep. Pulses of luteinizing hormone released by the pituitary gland at night wake us up and torture our rest hours. Unopposed estrogen can keep us awake and disrupt the natural sleep cycle.

Loss of Sex Drive

Human sexuality is a complex matter. The scientific and philosophical debate over the seat of sexuality has been raging for years. Is sexuality strictly confined to our physical plant, is it all mental, or is it a combination of mind and body? The inseparable connection between mind and body is clearly established by our hormones. When estrogen, progesterone, and testosterone levels are high, sexuality is at its peak. When the levels start decreasing in the forties and fifties, many women and men complain of decreasing libido, lack of sex drive.

For many women, vaginal dryness becomes a deterrent to active sexual intercourse. Vaginal dryness leads to painful intercourse; eventually, a vicious cycle develops in which the woman stops having sex, which only worsens the vaginal dryness. Sexual intercourse at any age improves the state of the vaginal lining. Stimulation of the vagina increases secretions and keeps the walls moist and responsive. With the decline of hormones and painful intercourse from lack of lubrication, women feel inadequate and unattractive. The situation may appear to be a localized problem, but it's systemic in origin. Correctly and effectively supplementing hormones relieves vaginal dryness, but good relationships, solid self-image, and an optimistic outlook on life guarantee successful maintenance of sexual drive.

A Word About Osteoporosis, Hypertension, High Cholesterol, Heart Disease, Cancer, Alzheimer's, and Other Chronic Illnesses

The new addition to the parade of problems caused by hormone imbalance after forty is the development of chronic illnesses. These are diseases of aging. They appear because our hormones are now dwindling; no mechanism for righting the balance of the hormones exists any longer. Our ovaries make little or no estrogen and progesterone regardless of how much our hypothalamus and pituitary glands demand it. Aging and the loss of estrogen and progesterone now turn symptoms into illnesses. Yet if we prevent the damage produced by the permanent loss of hormones, we can help prevent illnesses.

Osteoporosis

Estrogen stimulates bone production and inhibits the action of osteoclasts, the cells that destroy bone tissue. When the levels of estrogen diminish in later years, the positive effects of estrogen on the bone structure dwindle. Genetic predisposition to osteoporosis, taking anti-estrogen medications (tamoxifen, for example) or steroids (prednisone, for example) for serious medical problems, eating a diet poor in calcium and vitamin D, living a sedentary life, and avoiding sun exposure are all contributing factors to osteoporosis. When genetic makeup and age combine to increase the risk of osteoporosis, hormone supplementation, diet, and weight-bearing, strength-building exercises will help slow down the progression of this chronic illness.

Heart Disease

By the age of fifty, women catch up with men in the incidence of heart disease. Estrogen depletion is only one reason why. Genetics, smoking, obesity, lack of exercise, and high-animal-fat diets are contributing factors as well. Unfortunately, until ten years ago, no study had been undertaken to evaluate the effects of a deficiency of sex hormones on the female heart and establish a safe and successful program for prevention of heart disease in women. The PEPI trials, published in the *Journal of the American Medical Association* in 1999 and the *Archives of Internal Medicine,* were the first to look at the postmenopausal estrogen and progestin interventions. The results were interesting, yet not necessarily reassuring. Women who had been taking synthetic estrogen replacement therapy had a lower risk of getting heart disease only after years of therapy. For those women who took HRT for just a year, the risk of heart disease was the same as for women who did not take HRT at all. Presently, the Women's Health Initiative is still studying the effects of hormone replacement on the female heart. The results are contradictory. All we know is that statistically, women after fifty have the same incidence of heart disease as men. We can infer that there's a correlation between this fact and that women over fifty are in menopause and have low levels of estrogen and progesterone. While we are all waiting for research to be developed and studies created, I strongly believe that natural hormone supplementation, a heart-protective diet, exercise, and behavior modification techniques are beneficial in the fight against heart disease.

Alzheimer's

Estrogen depletion has been implicated in the increased incidence of Alzheimer's in older women. Estrogen's direct effect on the brain is stimulatory, while progesterone's is balancing and calming. Without the proper balance between estrogen and progesterone, deterioration of the brain can lead to Alzheimer's. The role of genetics, lifestyle issues, and diet can no longer be ignored. Recent studies in the *Archives of Internal Medicine* have raised questions about the role of estrogen supplementation in the progression of Alzheimer's. Some designer estrogens were evaluated to see if they might have beneficial effects on the brain. To date, studies have not conclusively demonstrated that designer estrogens prevent Alzheimer's.

Cancer

The aging process is intertwined with the development of chronic and often severe illnesses. Older women and men with low sex hormone levels have higher incidences of various forms of cancer. Before we jump to the conclusion that hormones cause cancer, though, let's remember that the pregnant woman with her very high levels of circulating hormones does not often get cancer. In fact, her hormones appear to provide her with protection from serious illnesses. Cancer's connection to hormones is under constant scrutiny from our medical community. Whether cancer in women is associated with synthetic hormone replacements is a source of heated debates. In chapter 9, I'll discuss studies relating to cancer and the use of synthetic hormones.

✣

We have now established two very important building blocks.

1. Hormone imbalances cause specific symptoms, and these symptoms are present and easily identifiable throughout our life. They aren't limited to menopause or premenopause.

2. From the first three chapters, we can now name these symptoms, correctly identify them when they appear, and connect them to the specific hormones that are out of balance.

In the next two chapters, I'll address the kinds of treatments available at present. I've chosen to break them down into conventional and alternative treatments. Although I believe you'll find that neither side offers the perfect solution, I want to give you a solid understanding to prepare you for what your physician may tell you, or what a health food store has to offer.

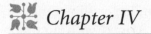

Chapter IV

Conventional Methods of Treatment for Symptoms of Hormonal Imbalance

$\mathcal{I}$ believe it's critical for you to know your options. My evaluation of current hormone imbalance treatments is based on both clinical and scientific information. Beyond my personal clinical experience, my staff and I have conducted a thorough and exhaustive research of the literature, both lay and professional.

A day doesn't go by that I don't hear women agonizing over treatment options for either menopause or symptoms of hormone imbalance in general. Conversations with new patients invariably sound like this:

"Doctor, I've done lots of research, gone online, read magazines and books on the topic of hormone replacement and menopause—and I'm lost. Most doctors offer either conventional, synthetic hormone replacement therapy or send you to the health food store for herbal remedies. I must admit to having tried practically everything, and nothing has really helped. I'm here because I'm at the end of my rope. Can you help me?"

Yes, I can.

Working with natural hormones has been like finding the Golden Fleece—the safe universal answer to symptoms of hormone imbalance. Before I share the solution, how I reached it, and how you too can easily find it, I want to address some of the other options you'll hear and read about. The reason you need to be familiar with alternative and conventional options is simple: Armed with accurate and broad-based information, you can be confident that when you make your decision, it's the best one for you.

Well-intentioned conventional doctors, friends, and holistic specialists are there to give advice. But all advice is biased. Given different information sources, educational backgrounds, and professional outlooks, no one can give you a complete overview of the different treatment options available in a thirty-minute session or over a cup of coffee.

The following two chapters contain a comprehensive overview of information on the most commonly used conventional and alternative options available for the treatment of symptoms of hormone imbalance. Use the information to take to your doctor and work together with him or her.

If you feel consistently better, stay with the program you've chosen; if you're dissatisfied with your results, move on to other options. Don't feel obligated to stay with only alternative or conventional therapies. Some women are afraid to mix therapies. Some women make alternative treatment choices based on TV ads, Internet information, and magazine articles. Most conventional choices come from physicians' offices. *However, no matter what path you follow, the best gauge of how your treatment works is how you feel.* I often see women who have been taking a particular type of medication for years and aren't feeling better. They're afraid to tell their doctors—and even to admit to themselves—that the medications aren't working. Remember, the goal is for you to feel better. In my experience, the real success stories come from people who truly integrate their therapies into their lives. There's a time and place for every type of therapy, and the key to success is to figure out how to combine them, when to take them, and for how long. You're entitled to try every option until you and your doctor find what works for you.

A word of caution before I enter the details of conventional therapies. Humans are works in progress. We are constantly changing—our bodies, our minds, and our tastes. If a remedy works today, it may not work tomorrow. You should not be wedded to one treatment. Learn to read the signs your body sends and listen to them. Your body will never lead you astray—ignoring its signals will.

The Side Effect Dilemma

The use of prescription medications to treat medical conditions invariably creates a high potential for undesirable drug side effects.

The Multiple-Adviser Problem

An outgrowth of our present health care system is that many people go to more than one doctor on a regular basis—conventional, alternative, and sometimes a combination of the two.

One physician no longer overlooks the care of the whole patient. No one supervises and coordinates all your medications, supplements, vitamins, diet, and exercise. Your health care in general is fragmented.

This situation shortchanges the patient, and renders the doctor potentially unable to truly help. Although it's difficult to accomplish, the burden is on you to make the doctor of your choice a true partner in your total health. If you can get organized, objective information, you can start helping yourself and your doctor put the puzzle together.

Look at migraines, for instance. Most medications used to treat migraines irritate your stomach, give you nausea, or leave you dizzy and vomiting. The side effects caused by the treatment of the migraine often will force you to take more medication.

And that's just the beginning. The medication you take to treat side effects has its own side effects, and so on.

Eventually, you realize that you cannot target a single symptom with one medication. No matter what you do, medications will affect multiple body functions and organs. It's like dropping a pebble into a lake—the ripple effect will be far reaching.

TREATMENT OPTIONS: CONVENTIONAL THERAPIES

Broken down by individual symptoms, here's a simple but functional list of conventional treatment options.

Acne

Topical medications are often the first line of treatment prescribed for teenage or middle-age acne. Commonly used prescription and over-the-counter creams, ointments, and washes include Benzaclin, Benzamycin, Cleocin T, Differin, Retin-A, and benzoyl peroxide. When topical treatments don't work well, most dermatologists prescribe Accutane. By law, dermatologists have to follow rigid guidelines in the use of Accutane. It can cause severe damage to unborn babies if taken while pregnant. Women of childbearing age should not take Accutane without taking birth control pills. The course of treatment is quite long, and liver function must be checked at frequent intervals in order to protect the patient from potential liver damage (also associated with the

Accutane treatment). Another potential side effect of Accutane is depression.

Bloating

Diuretics are the type of medications most frequently used to treat bloating, and are available by prescription only. Examples of the most commonly prescribed diuretics are Lasix (furosemide), Maxzide, and hydrochlorothiazide.

As with all medications, they should be used with caution, because their actions extend beyond their diuretic function. Diuretics can deplete your body of potassium and make you feel tired. I recommend that you take them with a potassium supplement or a banana, and don't use them for more than a couple of days in a row.

Postpartum Depression, Depression, and Mood Swings

Whether you're fifteen with mood swings, twenty-something with postpartum depression, or fifty and in the middle of a major depressive episode, the devastating effects of mood disorders cannot be overstated.

I often see women with successful careers, great parents, and devoted spouses who suddenly and without warning become overwhelmed and incapacitated by depression. These women are most likely to enter the medical system seeking help through their primary care physicians.

When a primary care physician, internist, or gynecologist sees a woman in the throes of depression, the knee-jerk reaction is often to start her on antidepressant medication and/or send her to a therapist.

If you're choosing the antidepressant route, find a psychiatrist—a specialist in the field of psychopharmacology. Use his or her expert help to decide on a medication to help improve your symptoms.

Antidepressants, used to treat women with depressive episodes, are prescription medications that work directly on the brain. The most popular ones increase circulating levels of serotonin, a member of a special class of hormones known as neurotransmitters.

Scientific data have established that people with high levels of serotonin in the brain feel better than those with low levels. Although no one knows exactly why this is the case, a whole series of antidepressants has been developed by the pharmaceutical companies. They are grouped under the heading of SSRIs—selective serotonin reuptake inhibitors. Their mode of action is to either increase serotonin release or inhibit serotonin metabolism, resulting in an overall increase in circulating serotonin levels.

Over the past ten years, antidepressants have become a staple in the field of psychiatry, where they seem to have become more popular than vitamins. Prozac is all too often referred to as vitamin P. Pharmaceutical representatives visit physicians' offices almost monthly with a new drug *du jour.* Prozac, Effexor, BuSpar, Wellbutrin, Zoloft, Paxil, Celexa, and Luvox are familiar names to all. For patients with anxiety and panic attacks, Valium, Xanax, Trazodone, and Ativan are commonly prescribed.

Older antidepressants belonging to a group called tricyclics include Imipramine and Desyrel. Their use has decreased since the advent of SSRIs. Beyond the good marketing for the SSRIs, often serious side effects have limited the use of tricyclics. Heart problems, palpitations, irregular beats, appetite increase, and sleep disorders are among the most common.

As for SSRIs, two of the most common side effects are lack of sex drive and weight gain. It isn't surprising that many patients discontinue the use of antidepressants due to side effects rather than to inadequacy of treatment.

Before you embark on a course of antidepressant medication, you might find it interesting to learn that a recent article in the *American Journal of Psychiatry* questions the effectiveness of antidepressant medications in actually relieving patients of their depressive symptoms.

I leave you with the following thought. If you're severely depressed, do see a psychiatrist and start medication. But speak with your doctor about using it only temporarily, to get you over the bad time. Work with your doctor to then discontinue its usage as soon as possible.

Hot Flashes

Hot flashes are the bane of any woman who has ever experienced them.

If I were to make a list of hormone imbalances' most annoying symptoms, hot flashes would be at the top, next to difficulty sleeping and loss of sex drive. Women will do practically anything to get rid of them.

Unfortunately, conventional medicine has two main options for treatment of hot flashes—synthetic hormone replacement and antidepressants.

The medical literature is unclear on how antidepressant medication works in the treatment of hot flashes. Research is virtually nonexistent. It appears the use of antidepressants is a desperate attempt to offer something to the patient in the absence of a real option, or a true understanding of the cause of hot flashes.

Of the hundreds of patients I have seen with hot flashes, not one has stayed with an antidepressant longer than a few months. The stories I hear are always the same. For the first few weeks, the medication seems to be helping, but then it stops and the doctor has to increase the dosage. With the increasing dosage, serious side effects may arise, while the flashes return and the patient—and often the doctor as well—just gives up. In my opinion, this is not a satisfactory method of combating one of the most troublesome symptoms of hormone imbalance.

Hot flashes are often treated with Premarin, Megace (in breast cancer patients), and occasionally birth control pills. All these medications are synthetic. Their alleged goal is to replace the low estrogen and progesterone levels believed to cause hot flashes. In my experience, if hot flashes are the only symptom a woman has, the side effects from these conventional therapies can be so numerous—and the level of dissatisfaction with the results so high—that they nullify any benefits.

While synthetic estrogens and birth control pills may eliminate hot flashes temporarily, in many women they can induce significant breast tenderness, vaginal bleeding, weight gain, mood swings, or gastrointestinal discomfort. Not to mention the question of a potential increase in the risk of breast, ovarian, and uterine cancer. (See chapter 9, Synthetic Hormones and Cancer.)

The controversy around synthetic estrogens in general makes the decision to take them to relieve hot flashes very difficult.

Insomnia and Sleep Disorders

Although insomnia and sleep disorders are often caused by hormone imbalance, other agents can be the culprits as well. Stress, change in environment, a bed partner who snores, shift work, jet lag, heavy exercise before bedtime, and drinking alcoholic or caffeinated beverages are all common causes of sleep problems. When a patient comes to the doctor's office and complains of insomnia, most physicians don't attempt to find the root cause of the problem. The doctor will usually take the easy way out and prescribe medications. Most sleeping pills belong to the group of medications called hypnotics (sleep inducing). The most commonly prescribed sleeping medications are Restoril, Ambien, Dalmane, Halcion, and Sonata. Another group of medications used to treat insomnia are benzodiazepines (also used to treat anxiety). They include Xanax, Valium, and Ativan. Over-the-counter medications that can be obtained without prescriptions include Excedrin PM, Extra-Strength Tylenol PM, Nytol, Sominex, and Unisom. These formulations contain diphenhydramine, an antihistamine that makes you drowsy.

Although sleeping pills do make you fall asleep, the quality of sleep they induce isn't natural. Users of these medications usually don't dream, and don't get the rest that natural sleep offers. REM (rapid-eye-movement) sleep is the most beneficial part of your sleep, and sleeping pills can eliminate it completely. As a result, people tend to be groggy the next day, walk around in a fog, and cannot concentrate; libido often disappears. Again, conventional doctors often don't treat the root cause of insomnia and sleep disorders. Unfortunately, this situation can lead people to become dependent on medication and never really address the reasons for their sleep problems. Over the past twenty-five years, I've written hundreds of prescriptions for sleeping pills, and I continue to do so today. If used judiciously, sparingly, and only when needed, sleeping pills can help with an occasional bout of insomnia in particularly stressful times. But if you find yourself taking them every night and still not feeling well rested, do stop and take stock.

Look at your life, your hormone status, and find the real reasons for your problem with sleep. (For more about sleep, see chapter 10.)

Headaches and Migraines

A visit to your internist or primary care practitioner with the complaint of headaches will usually elicit one of two reactions. Either the physician will perform an examination and, upon finding no abnormalities in your neurologic exam, treat you with medications; or he or she will send you to a neurologist for a battery of diagnostic tests to rule out everything from a brain tumor to multiple sclerosis. Assuming you get a clean bill of health and your diagnosis is migraines, the doctor will opt for medications. The most commonly used prescription medications to treat migraines are Imitrex (tablets and injectable), Fioricet, Depakote, and Inderal. Over-the-counter analgesics such as ibuprofen and acetaminophen are also prescribed. Narcotic painkillers like Percocet, Percodan, and codeine are occasionally used as well.

Most patients I treat for migraines respond well to Fioricet. As with all pharmaceuticals, the potential for side effects must always be considered. Stomach irritation, diarrhea, dizziness, fainting, and skin rashes are most common.

Over-the-counter medications include all the nonsteroidal antiinflammatories—Motrin, Aleve, Advil, and so on. They're all basically the same. Their chemical formulas and mode of action are extremely similar. Tylenol (acetaminophen) and all brands of aspirin (Bayer, Excedrin, and the like) are occasionally effective in treating mild migraines. If you're taking nonprescription medications and experience no significant improvement in your symptoms within twenty-four hours of taking them, go see a doctor. You may not necessarily have made the correct diagnosis and thus could be taking the wrong medication.

Loss of Sex Drive

Loss of sex drive in women is seldom addressed by conventional medicine and will require some potentially embarrassing and personal disclosures. To date, the only significant research in the area of sexual dysfunction was undertaken in the 1960s by Masters and Johnson. Human sexuality is such an important topic, it seems odd that all our information comes to us from thirty years ago. Sporadic articles appear in selected medical journals dealing exclusively with human sexuality, but as a rule these are not mainstream publications, and they're skewed toward the mechanics of male sexuality. The growing concern for treatment of male impotence led to the appearance of Viagra on the market in 1999. Viagra was created to improve erections in men, but it can help women as well. Its mechanism of action is to increase blood flow to the pelvic area, meaning penis or vagina. We need lots of blood flow to these areas to get aroused and have sex. Viagra does accomplish this, so from a mechanical standpoint this should be a panacea. Unfortunately, having sex and feeling sexy are not the same. Viagra may make sex mechanically possible but will do nothing for people whose flagging hormone levels make them lose all interest in sex.

For the women who are on synthetic hormone replacement (see chapter 6 for more on the difference between synthetic and natural hormones) or using topical vaginal estrogen, progesterone, or testosterone creams in the hope of improving their sex drive and vaginal moisture, be advised there is no proven scientific basis for these therapies. No data support significant improvement in sex drive for users of synthetic hormone replacement. To date, no study has been published addressing libido in aging women. The advice given to clinicians dealing with issues of sexuality in aging women found in publications of the American College of Physicians only skirts the issue. Unfortunately, it seems women's sexuality is still being swept under the carpet, because we have no real answers— and the medical profession appears to be afraid to address the questions. So doctors in clinical settings make most of their treatment decisions based on experience.

Testosterone, progesterone, or estrogen gels, as well as vaginal estradiol tablets, are being recommended by gynecologists. They work infrequently; the patients I see who have tried them invariably complain of the discomfort associated with having to insert creams and tablets in the vagina. Although they're administered locally and supposedly don't get absorbed systemically, no study has proven either their effectiveness or lack of systemic absorption. Vaginal dryness may be a local symptom, but its cause is systemic, and it should be addressed with systemic (meaning affecting the whole body) treatment.

In conclusion, conventional medicine may address some of your complaints from the standpoint of treatment with medications. Conventional medicine rarely addresses the root cause of symptoms, specifically in the area of hormone imbalance. Use this chapter as a starting point for your conversations with your doctor when addressing treatment in a conventional setting. Do not self-medicate. A good doctor–patient relationship will ensure the best outcome for you. So nurture a partnership with your doctor.

Chapter V

Alternative Treatments for Symptoms of Hormone Imbalance

Alternative therapies for hormone imbalance have emerged from the public's dissatisfaction with the limitations of conventional treatments. The conventional medical system's approach has mainly become one of diagnosing and treating disease rather than focusing on prevention. Although attempts to correct public perception have been made with a push for early diagnosis of disease, conventional medicine still seems to be of little help to healthy people who are simply looking for ways to stay healthy.

What conventional medicine considers prevention—Pap smears, mammograms, colonoscopies, cardiac stress tests—are actually methods of diagnosing diseases at early stages. Not one of these methods actually prevents diseases from occurring. Desperately aware of the need to prevent disease, the public has been searching for different avenues of true prevention. As our population lives longer and healthier lives, deferring the aging process has become a must for many people. In fact, a booming industry has developed in an attempt to satisfy this urgent need to stay young and healthy. Menopause and its attendant hormone imbalances have provided an enormous amount of fuel for the alternative health industry. Billions of dollars are spent every year by women in search of alternative help for symptoms of hormone imbalance, and millions of dollars are spent by the alternative industry on the development and promotion of alternative treatments.

While the alternative trend is booming, it behooves conventional doctors and patients to become vigilant, well informed, and careful in making safe and effective choices in this new area. In the past, many of my patients have come to me with questions on alternative therapies. As a conventional physician, I had limited access to the alternative world, and I had to do my own research. In the end, I became somewhat of an expert, and I've begun to use alternative therapies in my practice—with varying results. This chapter offers an overview of the alternative medicine world I've been sharing with my patients and have had some success with.

But before you try any of these remedies, I strongly suggest you seek professional advice. Do not follow advice given by salespeople in health food stores, or online advertising by marketers for the particular product they're selling. Do not fall prey to advertised specials for cure-all medications— you don't know what's in them, and you don't know what their effects will be. Find a physician interested in and experienced with alternative therapies. Even if these products are available over-the-counter, they may not be as safe as you think they are. Remember, there's only one of you; every time you take a supplement or medication, you're affecting your whole body's balance.

BE AN INFORMED CONSUMER

Regulation of Supplements and Herbs

The Food and Drug Administration is the federal regulatory body that approves medication use for the public. The purpose of the FDA is to assure that our foods and drug supplies are safe.

The process leading to FDA approval is very expensive, and it involves rigorous testing to prove effectiveness and substantiate claims. But FDA approval doesn't guarantee long-term safety. Even FDA approved medications have been taken off the market in a hurry when they proved dangerous to some users.

Many supplements and practically all herbs and other alternative therapies available over the counter are not regulated by the FDA. This does not necessarily mean that they aren't effective or safe. But it does leave the public in a precarious situation, since no federal watchdog agency is looking over many of the products we are buying in natural food stores.

Unfortunately, to make this situation worse, the information on natural product labels is often vague, and indications for usage are sometimes absent. You may never know exactly what's in the pill you're taking—and that's a scary thought.

So how do you choose which supplement or herb to take?

Who Is the Product Manufacturer?

When I started researching alternative treatments for symptoms of hormone imbalance, I learned something few people know: There are very few manufacturers of raw supplements, vitamins, and herbs. The enormous numbers of brands that fill the shelves of our health food stores are often the same product packaged by different companies.

Let me explain a little further.

Let's take dong quai—an herbal supplement that presumably improves hot flashes. Dong quai can be found in stores under as many as twenty different labels. Most is produced by a handful of manufacturing companies that package the raw herb under different labels. It's impossible to determine who the actual manufacturer is, or which product is better. Anybody can contract with a manufacturer, then get a packager, put their own label on a supplement, and then sell to the public. It's that simple. But again, it leaves the public in an uncomfortable position.

On the other hand, the industry has recognized the need for laboratory-tested brands, and a few manufacturers with long-standing solid track records have established themselves in the market. Their products are standardized. For the consumer, this is an important fact. *Standardized* means that the dosing is the same from batch to batch of supplement. For instance, St.-John's-wort is made by Pharmanex, and you'll find the same amount of active ingredients in every bottle of St.-John's-wort under the Pharmanex label. Since there is no regulatory agency that requires standardization of dosing, the manufacturer decides whether to provide internal testing and quality control for its products.

I advise you to stick with standardized labeled products for your own safety. Some examples of standardized labeled products include Pharmanex, Nature's Bounty, Solgar, and Twin Labs.

Bioavailability

Assuming that you've chosen a reliable brand with a proven track record, there still are no guarantees that a therapy will work for you. A stumbling block to benefiting the most from your chosen herb, vitamin, or supplement is bioavailability.

A big word with big implications, *bioavailability* refers to the amount of active ingredient in the medication or supplement that gets into your bloodstream and can be effectively used by your body. You could take pounds of supplements without visible improvement in your condition simply because your body is unable to extract their beneficial ingredients. A perfect example is yam in its natural forms. Although progesterone—a hormone our body needs—can be synthesized from fats and oils in yams, eating yams will never give us that progesterone. That's because our body can't make the progesterone in the yams bioavailable; we simply can't create progesterone from them. How the supplement gets into our system, what the body does with it once it's in our bloodstream, how much of it gets to our cells, and how they use it are only parts of the bioavailability story. When medications are tested for effectiveness, the most important marker is their bioavailability. With supplements and food substances that aren't under FDA scrutiny, bioavailability isn't even addressed, let alone tested.

Another example of variable bioavailability is calcium. Calcium is essential to good bone structure—but taking calcium supplements does not ensure that more calcium gets into our system, let alone into our bone cells or bones. Let's follow the path of a calcium pill you take in the evening, three hours after your last meal. Your stomach is empty, and the pill gets broken down into tiny components by gastric juices. If the components are small enough, the calcium supplement you took gets absorbed into your bloodstream. If they aren't small enough, these components go through the stomach, into the intestine, and out the other end—no calcium supplement for your body. If calcium does get absorbed into your bloodstream, it has a good chance of getting to your bone cells. But even once it's there, you have no guarantee that the cells that need the calcium have the enzymes, substrates, and all other necessary elements to absorb the calcium molecules and use them to make strong bones.

The fate of calcium in your body is similar to that of any other food or medication you take. There are lots of great supplements available with incredible potential benefits. The reason they don't live up to their promises is that they're not bioavailable. This is one of the key reasons many supplements just don't work.

In an attempt to improve bioavailability, many manufacturers advise taking their supplements on an empty
stomach. Hypothetically, a supplement is more likely to be
digested and absorbed by an empty stomach than if it were
mixed with other foods or medications. I stress the word
hypothetically, however, because there are no studies to substantiate the bioavailability of most supplements on the
market today.

Other methods of administration (besides pills and
tablets) have better rates of absorption and bioavailability.
Pharmaceutical companies have conducted numerous studies that confirm the better bioavailability of creams and gels.
The reason is primarily that skin is a more predictable
absorbent: It's the largest organ in the human body, and
blood flow to the skin is high in warm areas that blush such
as the chest, inner thighs, arms, and pulse points (wrists,
ankles, armpits, groin).

From a clinical standpoint, the degree of bioavailability
of a substance is directly proportionate to its expected effect.
If you're taking a pill to get rid of a headache and the
headache is gone thirty minutes to an hour after you took
the pill, clinically speaking, the pill was bioavailable enough
to be effective. When I discuss the bioavailability of natural
hormones or supplements, I'm referring to subjectively
measurable effects (elimination of hot flashes or night
sweats, for instance).

Professional Advice

When taking herbs and supplements, the type of professional advice you get is critical. Because herbs and supplements are not prescription medications, you can acquire
them without any supervision. That may feel like a freeing
experience, but the risk of getting into trouble and not even
knowing it is very high.

I'm blessed with a group of very intelligent and proactive patients. Whenever I ask them how they make their choices of supplements, the answers astound me—friends, TV ads, women's magazines, and the Internet. Missing from this list is the qualified expert—mostly because there aren't many experts. When you walk into a health food store, the salesperson behind the counter will most likely try to sell you the special of the day. When you go to alternative doctors or naturopaths, they will try to sell you their own products. Experts in alternative medicine don't know much about disease processes, and conventional doctors know little about herbs and supplements.

The following pages address alternative therapies for symptoms of hormone imbalance at a generic level. When it comes to brands, choose the tried and true—the brands that have been on the market the longest, are laboratory tested, and are found in reputable stores. Don't go for the bargains. They're usually of poor quality and a waste of money in the long run.

Until we have more integrative doctors—experts in alternative options who won't miss signs of disease and are willing to appropriately combine therapeutic options—the burden is on you to do the research. Gather all the information you can, and bring it to a physician willing to listen and work with you in the area of alternative treatments.

TREATMENT OPTIONS: ALTERNATIVE THERAPIES

Bloating

Herbal diuretics work almost as well as their prescription cousins. Their action is milder than their pharmaceutical counterparts, and they don't deplete your body's potassium as rapidly. Stomach discomfort does on occasion limit their use.

Chickweed, nettle, and uva-ursi are most commonly recommended for relief of water retention. The information on these herbs is scant and not based on data obtained from scientifically qualified studies. Their credibility comes from hundreds of years of use in herbal medicine practices. They can be purchased as capsules, powders, teas, and tablets. The dosing as well as the quality of the products depends on the particular manufacturer. Try a standardized laboratory-tested brand; if you obtain no relief after two or three uses, discontinue it and try another brand or remedy. My personal practice experience with diuretic herbs has been poor. I prefer a conventional diuretic because of its consistent action and the FDA standardization it carries.

Beyond its acceptability as a diuretic, uva-ursi herb has application as a urinary tract disinfectant, alleged to support the health of the urinary tract and kidneys. Clinical studies are limited and provide little information on the herb's effectiveness.

Nettle is a dual-action herb: Some herbal supplement distributors recommend nettle as a diuretic, while others suggest it be used for relief of allergies. No clinical references or scientific studies are published to date to substantiate either role for this herb.

Postpartum Depression, Depression, and Mood Swings

While there is no question that relaxation techniques, adequate sleep, and a diet low in refined sugars and processed, chemical-filled foods will help improve anyone's mood, there are a few herbal and other types of supplements that may help as well. Their value is that they are lower in cost and have fewer side effects than conventional antidepressants. No long-term clinical studies have yet been performed to compare dependency rates of conventional versus alternative antidepressants.

St.-John's-Wort

Extracts of this combination of herbs have long been used in folk medicine. In Germany, St.-John's-wort is licensed for the treatment of anxiety, depression, and sleep disorders. The extracts that make up this herbal remedy contain many different chemical classes, so the "active agent" is a matter of uncertainty. The use of St.-John's-wort extracts to treat mild to moderate depression is supported by more than twenty alternative clinical studies. Its efficacy is comparable to standard tricyclic antidepressants, but its side effects are less severe. Therapeutic response should be seen in days to weeks. A minimum treatment duration of four to six weeks for any significant response is needed. Side effects include fatigue, allergic reactions, and stomach discomfort.

SAMe

An amino acid supplement (not an herb), S-adenosyl-methionine *(ah-DEH-no-sil-meh-THY-o-neene)* has been used by some psychiatrists in the treatment of depression for the past twenty years, predominantly in Europe. Substantial claims for the use of SAMe in the treatment of osteoarthritis, liver disease, fibromyalgia, and chronic pain have been made in books published in the popular literature in the past two years. Because it's a supplement and doesn't require a prescription, it's easily accessible. Its alleged versatility made it very popular when information on it was first published. Unfortunately, while SAMe may have value in the treatment of mild depression, it fell short of the mark when patients in my practice tried it on their own. The problem with SAMe is that dosing is critical; unless taken under the supervision of a knowledgeable physician, results are usually poor, with the patient growing discouraged and discontinuing use. The over-the-counter recommended dosage for SAMe is much less than the therapeutic dosage needed for optimum results, making it potentially dangerous for a patient to self-medicate in order to reach the desired outcome.

I've had mixed results using alternative antidepressants in my practice. The cost of the medication often becomes prohibitive at the dose levels patients require to feel significant improvement in their symptoms. Thus, the use of conventional medications—covered by insurance—becomes more attractive. On the other hand, some patients have reported significant relief of temporary depressive episodes after taking SAMe or St.-John's-wort for periods of a few months. With St.-John's-wort, unfortunately, allergies are common enough to significantly limit its use. I selectively recommend taking either SAMe or St.-John's-wort for mild depressive episodes while balancing hormone levels for *short* periods of time—no longer than six months. The side effects of these alternative antidepressants are far less than those of prescription medications, and the addictive tendencies appear to be lower.

Hot Flashes

In chapter 4, I noted that conventional medicine has very little to offer with regard to the treatment of hot flashes. This isn't the case with alternative therapies. For approximately a year before natural hormones emerged as the best option for treatment of hot flashes, herbal supplements seemed the only viable possibility in my practice.

Vitex, black cohosh, and oil of evening primrose are the most popular herbal supplements in this category. Over the years, I've found that some women swear by these supplements, while others find them totally useless. You may find these herbs to work for a while, especially in younger women with occasional hot flashes. When hot flashes increase in frequency and other symptoms of hormone depletion compound the picture, however, herbal remedies rapidly become less effective.

Vitex

Also known as chasteberry, monk's pepper, agnus castus, agni casti fructus, and chaste tree, vitex has many active ingredients, including flavonoids and iridoids. Some clinical data exist to support the use of vitex extract in infertility associated with corpus luteum insufficiency, PMS and PMTS (premenstrual tension syndromes), acne especially associated with PMS, amenorrhea (lack of periods), polymenorrhea (too frequent periods), and mastodynia (breast discomfort). Most of the research on this product so far comes from Germany; results have led to the belief that vitex acts on the anterior pituitary, decreasing prolactin levels and increasing progesterone levels. Women with PMS have high levels of prolactin and lower-than-normal levels of progesterone. Vitex does improve the hormone balance, and thus may relieve the symptoms.

Although its use is widespread, vitex's side effects are quite limiting. They include diarrhea, weight gain, rashes, nausea, and headaches. Vitex should not be used in combination with hormone treatment or birth control pills, or while breast-feeding.

Black Cohosh

The primary application of black cohosh is to help ease the physical and mental changes associated with perimenopause and menopause—hot flashes, headaches, irritability, and depression. It has also been used to symptomatically treat hormonal deficits arising from ovariectomy and hysterectomy in younger women.

While some clinical studies do exist to support the primary application of black cohosh for the treatment of perimenopausal symptoms such as hot flashes, headaches, palpitations, ringing in the ears, sleep disturbances, and

Herbal Supplements and Soy Derivatives: A Word of Caution

*B*lack cohosh, isoflavones, ipriflavones, soy derivatives, soy milk, soy nuts, vitex, and dong quai are phytoestrogens. Their chemical makeup resembles human estrogen molecules closely enough for the body to misread them as estrogens. For this reason, they do alleviate some of the symptoms of estrogen deficiency. But they aren't estrogens, and they don't offer the beneficial effects we obtain from estriol or estradiol—natural estrogens. There are no research data to substantiate beneficial estrogenlike effects on the heart, bones, or brain.

Thus, while we think we're helping our situation by reducing the discomfort associated with our symptoms, we may be doing ourselves a disservice. Heart disease

mood disorders, its mode of action is poorly understood. Treatment requires at least eight weeks to alleviate symptoms. Clinical studies have ranged from eight weeks to six months, and the results are equivocal at best. Side effects include stomach irritation, nausea, and dizziness.

Although the literature in favor of black cohosh states that it can be used in conjunction with estrogen supplementation without side effects, I don't recommend this. Once on natural hormone supplementation, there's no reason to take additional supplements aimed at correcting the same symptoms.

and osteoporosis progress unimpeded when all we take are phytoestrogens.

A commonly used proof of the positive effects of soy comes from Japanese culture. Japanese women are known to suffer few if any side effects of menopause. The Japanese diet is rich in soy products—tofu, soy milk, and edamame—hence the popular connection between soy and problem-free menopause. No scientific data have substantiated this theory, however. Maybe Japanese women are genetically programmed to suffer fewer effects of hormone imbalance.

Until we have definite proof of soy's benefit to women, I don't recommend soy-derived supplements to my patients. I emphatically advise against isoflavones, ipriflavones, and genistein—all found in capsule, powder, and gelcap forms. This doesn't mean you should stay away from soy milk, tofu, or other soy products, though. Soy—in natural form and in moderation—is an excellent source of protein and should be used as such.

Oil of Evening Primrose

Classified as an essential nutrient, evening primrose contains essential fatty acids (EFAs), particularly omega-6 and gamma linoleic acid (GLA). Used for skin disorders and hyperactivity in children, evening primrose has found a great niche in women's health: PMS, breast health, pregnancy, and lactation. A study reported in *Lancet* in 1985 compared the effects of oil of evening primrose and two conventional medications on breast pain. Improvement of symptoms was not significant with oil of evening primrose, but there were fewer side effects than with conventional medications. Although often prescribed for symptoms of menopause, oil of evening primrose alone is of no value in the treatment of hot flashes. I must also caution that seizures have been reported in patients on antipsychotic medications who took oil of evening primrose with the medication (*Internal Medicine*, May 2001, "Alternatives Ease Some Menstrual Symptoms").

Insomnia and Sleep Disorders

Long before we had sleeping pills, herbal remedies and natural supplements were routinely used in the treatment of sleep disorders. These remedies are currently used for the treatment of insomnia not only in alternative practices, but in some conventional ones as well.

Valerian

Also known as vandalroot and garden heliotrope, valerian (an herb) finds its primary application in the treatment of insomnia and nervousness, as well as the improvement of sleep quality. A number of clinical trials have shown valerian to be an effective sedative for many people, with an efficacy comparable to standard prescription medications such as benzodiazepines (Valium). Valerian extracts generally cause fewer side effects than standard sleep medications, are better tolerated, and present a lower risk of dependency. Chronic use may result in headache, excitability, insomnia, and irregularities in the heartbeat.

Kava Kava

Used as a muscle relaxant and anti-anxiety herb, kava has a significant sedative component. It has been used safely in Polynesian society for centuries. In European phytomedicine, it's recommended for the treatment of mild insomnia, anxiety, and muscular tension. Some clinical studies have demonstrated that kava kava induces a state of relaxation and calm without interfering with cognition, memory, or alertness. Side effects are rare and associated with excess use. They include skin rashes and a syndrome—a collection of symptoms—similar to Parkinsonism. After discontinuation of the medication, the symptoms eventually disappear.

Melatonin

A normal secretion of the pineal gland, melatonin has captured the public's attention because of its alleged effects on mood, sleep, and jet lag. Promoted as a miracle cure, this supplement was the number one over-the-counter sleeping pill a couple of years ago. Unfortunately, its track record has not been so glorious. Study after study has failed to substantiate the claim that it's the ultimate natural sleeping remedy. Scientific and public health concerns over the dissonance between its wide use and evidence of benefit led to the convening of a workshop on melatonin by the National Institutes of Health in 1996. The workshop's general conclusions were that, while there have been no medical catastrophes caused by melatonin, no long-term positive effects have been identified, either. It might be of short-term benefit for insomniacs or travelers crossing multiple time zones, but that seems to be an individual opinion rather than a scientifically supported fact.

Headaches and Migraines

Alternative treatments for headaches include acupuncture, yoga, relaxation, visualization, massages, and aromatherapy. Many patients shy away from herbal remedies because of potential allergies that often worsen the headaches. Still, a few herbals have gained some acceptance in the treatment of headaches.

Dong Quai

Although its main application is in the treatment of menstrual disorders and menstrual cramps, dong quai is often used to treat headaches as well. While there are practically no clinical studies on this herb, animal and in vitro studies suggest that dong quai may be useful as an anti-inflammatory, smooth-muscle relaxant, analgesic, and mild sedative.

Feverfew

Feverfew is used in migraine prevention (prophylaxis) as well as treatment of migraines. The current consensus is that feverfew, an herbal supplement, may work prophylactically to prevent migraines, and that emphasis should be placed on the use of high-quality preparations with detectable and consistent levels of its key components (parthenolide levels of 0.2 to 0.9 percent). While clinical investigations have had mixed results, two studies indicate that feverfew treatment results in a reduction in frequency of migraines and milder migraines in pretreated individuals. Feverfew is also used in combination with vitamin B_{12} and magnesium with some decrease in frequency of headaches.

Side effects include stomach problems, diarrhea, allergic reactions to the fresh leaf when ingested, flatulence, and unpleasant taste.

Loss of Sex Drive

Alternative medicine comes up just as short as conventional medicine in the treatment of loss of sex drive experienced by most women as a result of hormone imbalance. The information we do have is anecdotal. It relates to the use of belladonna, an herb with central nervous system action. This herb induces dilation of the pupils and was used by courtesans in eighteenth-century Italy to attract men. I have never heard of it used in the twenty-first century for the improvement of sex drive. Today's pop culture brings to us Horny Goat Weed, testosterone herbs, and numerous other alternative remedies without any science behind them.

DHEA

Dihydroepiandrosterone is a precursor of estrone, testosterone, and estradiol. It's available over the counter and used as androgen replacement for women with loss of sex drive. The most popular products are Natrol and Just Right. Data on the efficacy of DHEA are variable. Improvement in sexual function may occur, but its side effects—increased hair growth and acne—limit its use.

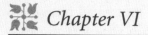 *Chapter VI*

$\mathcal{N}$atural Hormones

$\mathcal{A}$s symptoms of hormone imbalance start increasing, many women—whether in their teens or their sixties—react in a similar way. At first we try to ignore them: "I'm too young," we tell ourselves, or "this isn't really happening," or "it'll just pass." But when the symptoms become more intense and difficult to handle or new symptoms seem to appear every day, denial becomes impossible and we have to get help.

As I showed you in previous chapters, initially most women treat the individual symptoms. This approach is the result of advice from professionals and laypeople alike. At times, such treatment is successful. By taking this route, however, you reach a point where you could be taking up to thirty pills a day—medications, herbs, and supplements—with little or no success. How reasonable is this type of approach, and how long can anyone expect to stay with this treatment regimen?

Not very long.

And it's not just because there are so many pills to take, or because they're so expensive. No, above all, they often don't work effectively for many women. In this case, no matter how diligent you are in the research you do, how well you keep up with information, how organized you are in maintaining exercise, lifestyle, and diet routines, the results are often just not there. Whether you choose alternative or conventional therapies, or even integrate them both, stubborn symptoms may persist. This situation is untenable. And there is a better way.

I believe that the best treatment is natural hormones. I don't say this lightly. I've been caring for patients for decades, and I've suffered from the devastation of hormone deficiency myself. With respect to the patients I've cared for—and in myself—I've found that any other type of treatment except carefully and correctly administered natural hormones is not very effective on a long-term basis. In my experience, neither the conventional nor alternative therapies I've already discussed are as effective at restoring hormone balance. They may help alleviate symptoms temporarily, but if the root cause of the problems is hormone imbalance, measures that address only the individual symptoms will not be as helpful long-term.

For example, when hot flashes are treated with synthetic hormones, women may experience swollen tender breasts, have irregular periods with heavy bleeding, or migraines, or experience discomforting mood swings. Rather than effectively treating the root cause by taking hormone supplementation, the hormones the woman naturally produces are replaced with these synthetic substitutes, which introduce foreign substances to an already stressed system. My practice is full of stories of women desperate for help who found a satisfactory solution in natural hormones.

Georgia, for example, was thirty-four when she first came to see me. She had been going from doctor to doctor since she was eighteen. Her story was sad and all too common to me. When she turned fifteen, her period started—and with the beginning of her cycles, her life changed. She had terrible cramps, heavy bleeding, migraine headaches, severe bloating—and her periods were irregular to boot. Her mother took her to the family doctor. Ibuprofen for the cramps, a prescription medication to relieve headaches, and bed rest for the first day of her cycle was the doctor's advice. A few years later, Georgia, then a college student and frustrated by the constant nuisance created by her problems despite her good diet, exercise, and ibuprofen use, went to see a gynecologist. This time she had a workup: blood tests, a physical examination, and a pelvic ultrasound. As you might have guessed, all were normal. The doctor correctly diagnosed Georgia's problems as caused by hormone imbalance and recommended she take birth control pills. After six months on the pill her cramps were gone, her bleeding much lighter, but the migraines had become incapacitating, the bloating unbearable, the PMS unmanageable. Georgia went to headache specialists, endocrinologists, and even joined Weight Watchers. Nothing worked. After sixteen years of suffering, Georgia came to see me. I started her on natural hormones and, without exaggeration, her symptoms vanished within two months.

Vanessa came to me at the age of thirty-nine. She had a long traumatic history of hormone imbalance. Not unlike Georgia, she too experienced painful, heavy periods, migraines, and PMS. But Vanessa learned to live with them and never went to a doctor. When she entered her midthirties, however, her bleeding pattern became erratic and even heavier. She finally saw a gynecologist. An ultrasound taken in the doctor's office revealed a large fibroid in her uterus (a benign tumor whose existence has been associated with hormone imbalance). Vanessa was overwhelmed by the extensive bleeding and ensuing anemia. Her gynecologist suggested a hysterectomy and oophorectomy—and without much discussion, Vanessa agreed. She was almost forty and had no plans to have children, and she knew that women without children had a higher incidence of ovarian cancer, so why not get it all over with in one fell swoop? Lo and behold, shortly after the hysterectomy she started experiencing hot flashes, night sweats, weight gain, and severe depression. She was so desperate when she came to see me that she wanted her uterus and ovaries back—and her bad periods as well. Her doctor hadn't warned her of the disastrous consequences of removing the organs that manufacture the hormones we need to survive, and the devastation that hormone depletion would bring to her body and mind. I placed her on natural hormones. A few months after she started taking them, she did regain the hormone balance she could not live without. To this day, she's sorry she allowed the surgical procedure without exploring possible alternatives.

Connie was sixty-seven. She didn't even remember her last period. Her doctor had told her she didn't need to take medications to go through menopause. He was against synthetic hormone replacement, and while he thought soy and yam might help, he affirmed that everything else was useless. Connie braved it through the first five years of menopause, tolerating the hot flashes, the night sweats, and the loss of sex drive. But eventually she couldn't tolerate getting older—her bones were thinning, she became wrinkled, and her joints were stiff in the mornings. Her stomach problems abounded: Gas, heartburn, and weight gain became part of her everyday life. She grew depressed. She wanted more out of life; she wasn't ready to throw in the towel. I placed her on natural hormones and, by her sixty-eighth birthday, her friends wanted to know if she had had a face-lift, and what secret potion was giving her the energy she had so wonderfully regained.

The secret is natural hormones: a viable solution to problems caused by hormone imbalance, regardless of age. Not a miracle, not witchcraft, but a medical treatment that I've seen work time and again with my patients.

WHAT ARE NATURAL (BIOIDENTICAL) HORMONES?

Natural hormones are an FDA-approved class of products, mass-produced by pharmaceutical companies, and on the market for more than twenty years. They're called "natural" hormones and classified as bioidentical because their chemical formulas are identical in structure to the steroid sex hormones produced by our bodies.

Natural hormones are made from plants and mimic the chemical structure of the human hormone. Natural hormones are the closest in chemical structure, actions, and interaction to those hormones produced by humans.

The Effects of Natural Hormones on the Human Body

Because they're identical in structure to our own body's sex hormones, the action of natural hormones is relatively gentle, safe, and effective. Natural hormones attach themselves to *human cell receptors,* which are areas on the cell membrane that specifically recognize substances they need to use to maintain the body's health. Estrogen and progesterone receptors recognize natural hormones as their own.

Symptoms of hormone imbalance, as we get older, occur because of a deficiency, or lack of hormones in the body. This deficiency requires supplementation in order for the imbalance to be righted and symptoms to resolve. In our body, natural hormones act to directly target the root cause of hormone deficiency symptoms. Because they come from plants and have no synthetic molecules in their makeup, they don't compete with human hormone receptors. They *supplement* the action of human hormones, but don't displace or replace our own hormones from receptors on our cells. Thus, they don't compete with our own hormones.

The point bears repeating: Whether estrogens (estriol, estradiol, estrone) or progesterone, natural hormones do not interfere with, displace, or replace human hormones. Therefore, their action is gentle, and they are read by the human body as part of its own. Administered in a medically supervised manner, natural hormones can safely treat the root cause of hormone imbalances, deficiencies, and their attendant symptoms.

Natural Estrogen and Progesterone

Natural progesterone, commonly referred to as micronized progesterone, has the same chemical formula as the normally occurring sex steroid, progesterone, in humans. Short of human progesterone—which isn't presently available on the market—natural progesterone is the next best thing. Because its chemical formula is the same as the human progesterone, its actions are similar as well. Cellular receptors for progesterone recognize natural progesterone as the body's own and accept it. Any lack of endogenously produced progesterone can be effectively supplemented by natural progesterone—results are indeed remarkable.

Natural estrogen includes the same group of three hormones—estriol, estradiol, and estrone—as those made by the human body. Natural estrogens are made from soy. Their chemical formula is the same as the hormones manufactured by the human body. For this reason, they're known as bioidentical hormones. Just as with progesterone, natural estrogen is recognized by cellular receptors for estrogen as the body's own; thus, the supplementation offered by natural estrogens is easily accepted by the body. While natural hormones are derived from substances found in soy and yams, buying wild yam cream and other types of low-dose progesterone creams over the counter will *not* give you the benefits derived from natural hormones.

Many over-the-counter products include the words *natural* and *progesterone* on the label. These labels may confuse you. They do not have the same concentrations as the natural estrogen and progesterone I'm referring to in this chapter. Our body doesn't have the enzymes and chemical pathways necessary to transform soy or yams from their natural forms into usable hormones. (See chapter 5 for more information on phytoestrogens and bioavailability.) The active molecules of estrogen in soy, and progesterone in yams, cannot be utilized by our body directly from the raw materials. If you buy yam cream and put it on your skin, the progesterone in the cream isn't bioavailable to your body—the human system cannot effectively process that cream and transform it into the progesterone it so desperately needs.

The same is true for soy. Any soy product we eat cannot be transformed into real estrogen we can use. Only by special processing in pharmaceutical laboratories can the active hormones be synthesized from soy and yams—and only in this highly refined form can our bodies take advantage of the estrogens in soy and the progesterone in yams.

THE DIFFERENCE BETWEEN
SYNTHETIC AND NATURAL HORMONES

In chapter 4, I addressed conventional medical treatments for individual symptoms of hormone deficiency or imbalance. When hot flashes, irregular periods, and menopause occur, many physicians turn to synthetic estrogens.

To make safe and well-informed choices, you need a clear understanding of the differences between natural and synthetic hormones.

Synthetic Hormones

Whether estrogen (Premarin, Estratab, Ogen, and so on—see chapter 9) or progesterone (medroxyprogesterone, Provera, progestins, and the like—see chapter 9) look-alikes, synthetic hormones are all foreign or synthetic substances processed and manufactured from chemicals or animal products in a laboratory. They bear little resemblance to hormones our bodies naturally make. The reason they alleviate some of our symptoms is that our cells misread certain portions of the molecular structure of these substances. They are chemical hybrids. If you're currently on HRT prescribed by your conventional doctor, you may be taking one of these synthetic hormones—and may not be getting the results you need. The synthetic hormones replace your own hormones with foreign molecules rather than supplementing or balancing them—which is the mode of action that may best help your condition.

How Synthetic Hormones Were Developed

Organically foreign, synthetic estrogens are derived from pregnant mare's urine. The choice to use animal-source estrogen was made by pharmaceutical companies more than thirty years ago. At that time, it made sense in a field that had just come into existence. Insulin, another important hormone, was developed at that time. When pork and beef insulin came to the market, they saved the lives of many children with juvenile diabetes.

The enormous success of insulin opened the door for the development of other animal-based hormones. At the same time, estrogen from pregnant mare's urine was being created. However, the use of pork and beef insulin was more widespread and serious side effects were surfacing. Rapidly progressive kidney disease and blindness has been associated with the use of animal-derived insulin. This is what motivated the development of human insulin. Once human insulin arrived on the market, we rarely heard of beef and pork insulin again or their significant side effects.

Unfortunately, this was not the case with sex hormones. Estrogen derived from pregnant horse urine came into existence in the 1950s. Since then, it has remained the main source of estrogens made by pharmaceutical companies recommended for the treatment of menopausal symptoms. Because its use was not very extensive in the early stages, little was learned about potential side effects arising from the use of synthetic estrogen. There seemed to be no problems.

You should know that the chemical composition of synthetic estrogen is different from that of natural hormones. Because it's derived from horses, it's not the same as human estrogen. Although it contains the estriol, estrone, and estradiol found in the human estrogen molecule, it also contains equilin, an additional estrogen molecule specific to the horse.

Questions on how equilin affects estrogen receptors in humans abound. Does equilin create its own new receptors on human cells? Does equilin displace human estrogen from its own receptors? Does our immune system see equilin as foreign and react against it by making us sick? Scientists haven't definitively answered these questions because pharmaceutical companies have little vested interest in finding out. In the meantime, the women in need of hormones are left without complete and factual information.

Progestin

Progestin is the synthetic, not-found-in-nature progesterone. In my opinion, even to call it "progesterone" is misleading. The molecular structure of progestins is unlike that of progesterone. Progestin's chemical makeup may loosely resemble natural progesterone, but it won't achieve the same results.

Progestin was developed to compensate for a dangerous side effect associated with the use of unopposed synthetic estrogen: increased incidence of endometrial (lining of the uterus, also called uterine) cancer. Progestin was created in the 1970s when the dangers of synthetic estrogen replacement were first published in the medical literature. So if you're presently taking synthetic estrogens (ERT), your doctor may have you taking progestins (Provera, for example) to offset those dangers. Progestin is used in combination with synthetic estrogens in the hope of diminishing the dangers posed by the use of unopposed synthetic estrogens (see chapter 9).

To date, progestins (also known as progestagens) have not proven to be of any independent value to the patient. Used alone without estrogens, progestin can induce heavy vaginal bleeding and depression.

It is of the utmost importance to avoid confusing progestin with natural progesterone. Progestin is a chemically altered, not a naturally occurring, hormone. Progesterone is the natural hormone our body makes to balance the unchecked action of estrogen. Natural progesterone, synthesized from yams and soy beans, is the substance closest to our own body's progesterone. Progesterone is safe and absolutely necessary to our well-being. Progestin is not. While progestins should not be used alone, natural progesterone can and is often used alone. Its use is safe and does not induce dangerous side effects.

NATURAL HORMONES AND THE CONSUMER

Natural hormones are only available for sale in bulk—large powder-filled drums, produced by the manufacturers of raw pharmaceutical products. The manufacturer sells the raw natural progesterone, estriol, estradiol, and estrone in generic form directly to small compounding pharmacies or large pharmaceutical companies. From this point, the pharmacy staff prepares the final product for distribution directly to the public. The final product is either a rigidly dosed pharmaceutical medication (see Available Hormone Preparations, p. 213) or an individualized made-to-order compound.

Prometrium is an example of the former—a branded tablet form of rigidly dosed, natural progesterone mixed in a peanut oil base, produced by a large pharmaceutical company and distributed by prescription to the public through most retail pharmacies. It is the only commercially available natural progesterone in tablet form.

Monica is fifty-seven and has been seeing me for two years. She has been very happy with natural hormones. Because she lives a good distance away from my office, she continues to see her gynecologist for annual physicals and Pap smears. When Monica started going through the menopausal transition, she asked her doctor what to do. The doctor prescribed a synthetic estrogen and progestin and sent her on her way. Monica did not do well with this synthetic regimen. She called her doctor and asked about natural hormones. Her doctor told her that they don't work, and directed her to stay on the synthetics. Dissatisfied with this answer, Monica came to see me. After about a month on natural hormones she reported that she felt great, but said that she never told her doctor she switched. To this day, her doctor believes she's taking synthetic hormones and doing beautifully on them. Instead, she takes natural hormones without sharing that information. Unfortunately, I know too many Monicas. This situation is almost tragic. It's a poor reflection on the communication between doctor and patient, and it keeps information about the efficacy of natural hormones away from doctors. It also may prevent more women from having access to natural hormones.

WHY HASN'T YOUR CONVENTIONAL DOCTOR TOLD YOU ABOUT NATURAL HORMONES?

Although most doctors are aware of the existence of natural hormones, few know what to do with them. Most physicians in clinical practice get their information about the medications they prescribe from three sources: pharmaceutical representatives, continuing medical education courses, and medical trade journals. Pharmaceutical representatives regularly visit doctors' offices to offer samples of their newest products. Along with the free samples, they distribute scientific articles on the medications they're promoting, indicating how effective their featured medications are. When evaluating these medications, doctors must keep in mind that the manufacturer of the product likely sponsored the referenced research.

The above scenario also occurs in continuing medical education courses and articles published in medical journals. An inordinately large portion of medical information reaches doctors courtesy of pharmaceutical companies. When a study is conducted and paid for by the company that stands to benefit from the studies' positive results, doctors must ask themselves how objective the research is.

Pharmaceutical companies spend millions of dollars on publicity for their patented medications, because patented medications bring the highest revenues. A medication can be patented only if its chemical structure is novel. Synthetic compounds, foreign to the human body and manufactured in a lab, can be granted patents. Exclusive market share and millions of dollars in sales are practically guaranteed to the pharmaceutical company that holds the patent on a widely prescribed medication. In order to secure this market share, pharmaceutical companies will work hard to protect their patented products.

Because natural hormones are found in nature, their chemical formulas are not novel. Thus, pharmaceutical companies currently have little interest in researching, developing, or promoting them. Instead, pharmaceutical companies chemically alter the progesterone molecule to produce a patentable progesterone-like substance called progestin. As a result, the best (and almost the only) way for consumers and doctors to hear about the significant benefits of natural hormones is word of mouth. Although this creates more gradual recognition, such promotion should not be underestimated. After all, the proof is in the pudding. Natural hormones, in my experience, are more effective and safer than any other treatment I've seen or used for symptoms of hormone imbalance. Virtually none of my patients who start natural hormones ever turns back to synthetics!

NATURAL HORMONES ARE THE SOLUTION

After many years of getting poor or no results with conventional HRT (synthetic hormone replacement) in my practice, the chance to offer my patients natural hormones came as a miracle. The medical literature hints at the existence of natural hormones and their beneficial effects. However, there are no programs or outlines of any particular method of distribution that a physician can follow when he or she wants to prescribe natural hormones. These circumstances make it very difficult for the average clinician to provide adequate advice and monitoring for patients who want to take natural hormones. This situation forced me to build my own program and to write *The Hormone Solution*.

When Ellen came to see me, she was in her early forties. The first time I saw her, I was not yet prescribing only natural hormones in my practice. Ellen had complaints of weight gain, a change in her periods, and stomach problems. A thorough examination and gastrointestinal workup failed to uncover illness in Ellen. Together, we decided to try Ellen on birth control pills. Scientific data encouraging the use of birth control pills in perimenopausal women abounded and came almost exclusively from Europe. After three months on birth control pills, Ellen returned to my office in tears. She felt worse. Her breasts had ballooned, her sex drive disappeared, the migraines had worsened, and her mood was foul. She was miserable with the results and wanted something else. I decided to try natural hormones.

Miraculously, Ellen's symptoms began to disappear; she was her old self in just two weeks' time.

Ellen was a turning point for me. The effectiveness and superiority of natural hormones did not go unnoticed in my practice.

Laura, another patient of mine, was sixteen and had severe PMS and cramps that incapacitated her every month. Her mother took her to a gynecologist, who wanted to put Laura on birth control pills. Her mother was concerned and brought Laura to me. In the past, I would have advised Laura to go on birth control pills as well. By this time, however, my success with natural hormones had been so great that I didn't. I instead started her on natural progesterone for two weeks before her period. Within two months, the cramps and PMS were gone. And unlike most of my other patients who were taking birth control pills, Laura didn't gain weight.

In a few months' time, I found myself changing from a conventional doctor—who depended upon synthetic hormones to treat these problems—to one who switched all patients with hormone imbalances to natural hormones. The results were remarkable. I could treat each patient as an individual because I could fine-tune the amounts of hormones I used. No prior experience in my medical practice offered such satisfaction or success. Guided by my conventional medical training and experience, I gathered information by using evidence-based medicine and by reviewing available data from scientific journals on natural hormones. The program I developed has worked to effectively address symptoms. Ellen, Laura, and I may have pioneered the program, but soon thereafter many others followed. And to this day (five years later), I'm not aware of anyone I've treated who has returned to synthetic hormones.

Natural Hormones Are Available by Prescription Only

Natural hormones, in the strength that provides significant symptom relief, can only be obtained by prescription, and unfortunately this has limited their use. Without access to a lot of information and clinical data on natural hormones, doctors have difficulty learning about their merits and becoming knowledgeable in methods of usage. Without adequate sponsorship for research, the scientific data on

What About Over-the-Counter Preparations?

It's common to see the term *natural hormone* on labels for over-the-counter products with low concentrations of natural hormones. As a result, you may mistakenly believe that you have retail access to the same concentrations as those available by prescription only. The concentration of over-the-counter natural hormones and the means by which they're administered don't have the same benefits as the natural hormones your doctor can prescribe.

It's sad but true: Such products can be a waste of time and money. If all you need is a little hormone supplementation, try them, but if you feel no better after using them for a few weeks, speak with your doctor about the natural hormones available by prescription only.

natural hormones is not easily available to the physicians who can write the prescriptions.

Sadly, few physicians take the time and the expense to build a solid natural hormone practice. This situation does an enormous disservice to doctors who want to help their patients feel better, and women who are desperately searching for relief.

HOW CAN YOU GET NATURAL HORMONES?

To get natural hormones, you have to ask your doctor to write a prescription, then find a pharmacy to fill it. This is

What's the Pharmacy's Role?

Prescription-quality natural hormones are specifically mixed in compounding pharmacies. According to the New York State Board of Pharmacy, any regularly licensed pharmacy can add *compounding* to its list of services. Other states have different rules, but in general, once licensed by the state board of pharmacy, any pharmacy can technically mix medication per doctor's orders. No special licensing requirement exists to distinguish between a compounding pharmacy and what the public recognizes as a regular retail pharmacy.

Lists of compounding pharmacies specializing in filling prescriptions for natural hormones are usually found at the end of consumer books on menopause and alternative treatments. These are regular pharmacies that have developed among their other areas of services an expertise in natural hormones. Since regular pharmacies

the first and only stumbling block in the process of getting natural hormones. How do you find a doctor who will write the prescription, or how do you convince your present doctor to do it?

The first step toward getting yourself on natural hormones is to open the lines of communication with your doctor. He or she may already know something about them, or may be willing to find out more. He or she can write a prescription and help you get it filled. If your doctor isn't receptive, ask why and consult other doctors in your area who may use natural hormones. If you have no luck, I have included a Resources section at the end of this book that

don't have facilities for or interest in filling natural hormone prescriptions, compounding pharmacies arose to fill the need. But remember, natural hormones in therapeutic doses (amounts that can actually help us) require a physician's prescription.

Natural hormones must be individually prepared, and because the only standardized product in a compounded formulation is the natural hormone, you need a pharmacist who specializes in such formulation, to work under the supervision of a physician who is knowledgeable in the dosing and methods of administration of natural hormones.

The pharmacy should only be there to fill the prescription to your physician's specifications. You must find an educated physician or suggest your physician review the Hormone Solution Program. (Also see Available Hormone Preparations—a chart—at the end of this book.)

lists my Web site—www.HormoneSolution.com—where you can find a listing of doctors who work with natural hormones. I have also included information on the Natural Hormone Pharmacy (the only compounding pharmacy in the country specializing exclusively in natural hormones) and the 800 number you and your doctor can use to get more information. You are no longer alone!

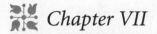

Chapter VII

The Hormone Solution Program and Dosage Guidelines

*W*hen I first decided to try natural hormones, I went to my local pharmacist with the prescription I had written after doing research for six months. He was very helpful and prepared natural micronized progesterone and estradiol powder in capsules. The improvement in my own symptoms was remarkable. Within days, my night sweats and hot flashes were gone, and my mood was even again. I had found my miracle cure and started ordering the same for my patients.

After a few months, however, some of my patients and I noticed that the hormones worked inconsistently. If we took the capsules on a full stomach, were stressed, had a virus or other illness, or took other medications, the hormones didn't work as well. After a couple of attempts at changing dosages and types of capsules, I realized that the problem came from the unpredictability of absorption of the capsules. If the hormones were absorbed, we felt good; if not, the symptoms returned. Remember the issue of bioavailability? This was a perfect experiment in the bioavailability of natural hormones. I had to find another, more reliable route of getting the hormones into our systems. The question was not if they worked, but rather how to ensure that they got into our bloodstreams consistently. The way I determined whether the hormones were in fact absorbed was very simple—we felt better.

To find the best method for absorption of medication, I researched the pharmaceutical literature. The result of my search was that *transdermal preparations*—creams and gels containing active medications applied to the skin—display a high degree of bioavailability. This means that they are absorbed the best by the body. When hormones are placed in transdermal creams, they are applied directly to the skin of the neck and upper chest. Areas that blush have good blood flow and are ideal for application of creams. Absorption occurs rapidly when the cream is gently rubbed into the skin. The incidence of allergic skin reactions appears to be negligible. Because creams are so well absorbed, small doses of hormones can be used. There are other benefits from transdermal creams; absorption through the skin bypasses the first pass through the liver, thus minimizing stress to liver function. Transdermal administration facilitates the direct absorption of the active ingredients, thus avoiding side effects to the gastrointestinal tract following oral intake.

My helpful local pharmacist could not provide the laboratory facilities necessary to create the best transdermal preparation for my natural hormones. He did help me locate a pharmacy with the necessary facilities, however. So I ordered my hormones from a compounding pharmacy in California. Although they were expensive, I was willing to try them for a while. I felt wonderful. The patients who could afford them and ordered them with me felt great as well. Three months after beginning to use transdermal creams, I had finally found consistency in action.

But there were two hitches—the price and the method of administration. You needed a Ph.D. in chemistry to be able to figure out how much to take to get the amount prescribed. If I had such a hard time myself, I wondered how a layperson with no medical background would do. I felt I had no choice: I had to figure out on my own how to make the cream form user friendly and financially accessible—and see whether insurance reimbursement was possible for my patients. Three years later, having invested significant financial and professional resources, I was able to formulate a transdermal preparation of natural hormones that met these

*W*hile a thorough review of conventional and alternative medical literature reveals little on the use of natural hormones, there's some comprehensive information in publications like *Natural Pharmacy, Compounding Pharmacy,* and in books by Dr. John Lee, MD, including *What Your Doctor May* Not *Tell You About Menopause,* along with *The Natural Hormone Replacement* by Johnathan Wright, MD, and numerous other consumer books on menopause.

The reason natural hormone therapy isn't a popular subject of conventional medical studies is that its large-scale use is limited by the need to individually adjust the dosage. It's still a cottage industry, but one whose success has become too important to ignore. In the instances when evaluations of the usage of estradiol or micronized progesterone find their way into the medical literature, the results are invariably positive. (See References.) Data substantiated by clinicians working with natural hormones at Vanderbilt University and women's clinics in California, Arizona, Florida, and Washington reinforce the positive results of natural hormone supplementation.

standards that could be used by pharmacies and guide doctors as they treated patients. Other doctors who specialize in
natural hormones have done the same.

METHODS OF NATURAL HORMONE ADMINISTRATION

High on the list of benefits to users of natural hormones
is the flexibility in dosing and the opportunity for user-
friendly methods of administration. This flexibility allows
your physician to fine-tune your treatment to reach your
ideal individual goals.

Natural progesterone, estriol, estrone, and estradiol can be
dispensed in capsules, tablets, gelcaps, creams, and sublingual
troches. Estriol, estradiol, and estrone can also be combined.
The combination of estriol and estradiol is branded Biest.
Estriol, estrone, and estradiol are branded Triest.

Transdermal creams are quickly becoming the leaders.
Not only is the product easy to administer, but the method
ensures more precise dosing, excellent absorption, and the
flexibility to tailor each dose to each individual patient's
needs. In my extensive practice, my colleagues and I have
found that transdermal formulations offer the best absorption, using the least amount of hormones per dose. Still,
your own doctor's ability to offer you totally individualized
therapy with natural hormones depends on his or her level
of comfort and experience with the therapy.

I find many doctors I speak to are in a quandary. They
want to help their patients, but they have nowhere to turn.
Synthetic hormone replacement is the only form in which
hormones are currently mass-marketed. Most doctors are
aware that patients are afraid to use them because of their
side effects and association with increased risk of cancer. But

many doctors are missing the information on natural hormones they need to prescribe them to their patients.

Some doctors thus hedge their bets. They will tell you natural hormones don't work—that not enough data are available—when in fact all they need is the information on how to prescribe these hormones and where to order them. I encourage you to take this book, and any other literature on natural hormones you can find, to your doctor and begin a discussion on natural hormone supplementation. In order to make it easier for your doctor to start working with natural hormones, I have included in this chapter my general guidelines for doses and combinations of hormones, which can serve as a starting point for your physician as he/she considers your specific medical history and condition and tailors the treatment to your needs and symptoms.

THE HORMONE SUPPLEMENTATION PROGRAM

My experience has shown that most people fit into one of five groups, according to age and symptoms. Beyond the basic groupings, I have found it necessary to adjust the preparations in order to meet individual patient needs in approximately 10 percent of patients.

Work with your physician to see whether you fall into one of the groups I've identified through my years of experience with this treatment. Undergoing a thorough examination by your physician and then discussing your symptoms will help ensure proper and successful treatment for you. If you belong in the age group identified and experience a minimum of two of the symptoms mentioned, you may well experience remarkable benefits from trying the natural hormone program indicated.

GROUP I:
PRELIMINARY SUPPLEMENTATION
Age Group:
Teens and early twenties

Symptoms:
> Acne
> Mood swings
> Stress syndromes
> Occasional night sweats
> PMS
> Occasional sleep disturbance

Menstrual Status: Normal cycles

Remember Michelle, the fourteen-year-old with acne from chapter 3?

Michelle's mother brought her to me at the end of her rope. Reluctant to allow the dermatologist to start her on the drug Accutane, which has some potentially serious side effects, to treat her acne, her mother chose to try my program for Michelle. We gave Michelle topical antibiotics and progesterone cream. Six months later, Michelle was free of acne and has been a patient in my practice for the past two years with no further problems.

Louise, the seventeen-year-old with the severe mood swings, saw a therapist and was started on a prescription antidepressant before she came to me. I saw her, started her on a micronized progesterone program, and helped her change her diet and sleep patterns. Within three months, Louise was able to stop taking the antidepressant. Now, three years later, she has had no problems with her moods, and she is still on micronized progesterone when needed.

There are months she goes without the aid of the progesterone because her body is able to balance her hormone needs itself. She has learned to read her body's messages and use progesterone only if necessary.

Natural Hormone Supplementation Guidelines

Micronized progesterone in transdermal cream, 4–6 mg/kg of body weight per day. The cream is applied to the neck, upper chest, and inner wrists, as convenient. If you have acne, don't rub on your face.

Administer, generally, from two weeks before the onset of menses to the whole month, depending on symptoms. Before starting on progesterone cream, topical treatments as described in chapter 3 may be attempted in patients with acne alone. From experience, I find that when a detailed and reliable history is obtained, more than one symptom exists. When this is the case, progesterone cream can address the root cause of the symptoms and reestablish the hormone balance.

GROUP II:
ADULT SUPPLEMENTATION
Age Group: *Midtwenties through thirties*

Symptoms:

PMS	Breast tenderness
Bloating	Food cravings
Migraines	Occasional depression
Decreasing attention span	

Menstrual Status: Normal menses

Remember Marcia, the twenty-five-year-old with postpartum depression?

She was correctly diagnosed by her psychiatrist,

but the treatment he offered was not what Marcia wanted. She wasn't willing to sacrifice her sex life and trim body to the antidepressant medication the doctor proposed and its side effects. She came to my office, and I started her on a combination program of estradiol and micronized progesterone that mimicked her normal cycle. It increased the estrogen and progesterone levels that were dropping too fast after the birth of her baby. The drop in estrogen had precipitated the drop in serotonin that directly affected her sense of well-being, and the drop in progesterone affected her sense of calm. Once supplemented with the natural hormones, Marcia did not need to take antidepressants. She recovered from her postpartum depression within a few months. After the birth of her second child, two years later, Marcia took the combination of natural hormone creams prophylactically for six months and did not experience another episode of depression.

Hormone Supplementation Guidelines

Micronized progesterone in transdermal cream, 4–6 mg/kg of body weight per day of use.

Estradiol, 0.006–0.008 mg/kg of body weight per day of use.

The creams are applied to the upper chest and lower neck areas, inner arms or wrists—areas that are warm and have good circulation and thus enhanced absorption. The dose is generally cycled to follow the woman's natural cycle for a minimum of three months and a maximum of one year, based on the correlation to symptoms.

Often, patients ask what they should do if the symptoms stop. I often advise them to continue taking the hormones, because it's likely the reason symptoms stopped is that the hormones are working. Sometimes I advise a patient to stop taking the hormones for a few weeks and see what happens. If she stays well, there may be no reason to continue; if the symptoms return, she can always start the hormones again. The beauty of natural hormones is that there generally are no adverse effects if they're suspended or reintroduced.

GROUP III:
PREMENOPAUSE
Age Group: Thirty-five to forty-plus

Symptoms:

Acne	Hair loss
Mood swings	Digestive problems
Sleep disorders	Hot flashes
Bloating	Night sweats
Migraines	Depression and anxiety
Weight gain	

Menstrual Status: Menses may or may not be regular

Olga, the thirty-five-year-old we met in chapter 3, belongs in this group. She had severe bloating, PMS, and sore breasts. She thought she was mentally ill. Her life was falling apart, and doctors couldn't help her. She was told she was premenopausal, perimenopausal, and sometimes none of the above. Because she was thirty-five, she was too young for any of these labels; she was having periods, and that precluded conventional doctors from treating her with hormones (the general rule in conventional medicine is that you don't start HRT before menstruating stops); and alternatives didn't work. She had no definitive diagnosis; she found no helpful solutions. When I saw her, I didn't give her a label—

creating a diagnosis was of little importance. I just wanted to help her feel better. All the blood tests, X rays, and examinations performed had been normal. Her prior physician had done a great job of testing her to rule out medical problems. I was fortunate to come in on her case knowing that her problems were caused by decreasing levels of estrogen and progesterone. Her physician could make this diagnosis, but could not offer the treatment. It was the loss of the cyclic function of the hormones and the inability of her body to make up for the imbalance that needed correcting. All I had to do was give her back the missing hormones and balance their levels to mimic what used to be her personal normal cycle.

There was only one option I felt would work. I placed her on natural hormone supplementation. And she returned to her old self within two months. That was four years ago. Now, she's still on natural hormones; only her combinations have changed, to fit her changing needs.

Hormone Supplementation Guidelines

Micronized progesterone, 4–6 mg/kg of body weight per day of therapy.

Estradiol, 0.007–0.009 mg/kg of body weight per day of therapy.

The dose is generally cycled with changing concentrations of these combinations based on the woman's cycle or desire to stop the cycle. The length of time a woman takes a particular hormone combination usually depends on how she feels. I find that with the passage of time, most of my patients move on to the following level of therapy. Changing the combinations of hormones a woman needs is usually brought on by a conversation between patient and doctor.

The goal is to always help the woman feel her best. Blood tests are of little value (see chapter 8) when dealing with specific symptoms. If the combination of hormones is correct and the method of administration bioavailable, the results are remarkable. Adjustment of dosage is easily accomplished with the patient's cooperation. I find that once women start feeling better, they become excellent partners in their own care. They invariably help the doctor find the ideal hormone combination for themselves. My advice to the doctors who follow my Hormone Solution Program protocols is to listen to the patients; they will always guide us well.

GROUP IV:
PERIMENOPAUSAL
Age: Forty to fifty-five

Symptoms:

Mood swings	Sleep disorders
Bloating	Migraines
Weight gain	Hair loss
Digestive problems	Hot flashes
Night sweats	Depression and anxiety
Loss of sex drive	

Menstrual Status: Irregular to cessation

This is the group where all hell breaks loose. I belong in here. Conventional medications might treat some of the symptoms, as you know from chapter 4. Alternative options might work for a while, as we learned from chapter 5. Going on birth control pills or synthetic estrogens is the typical option conventional medical practice offers. The diagnosis your physician is making is correct. You've been identified as suffering from hormone imbalance. You've experienced all the symptoms and are getting more and more panicky about what to do and where to turn.

Natural hormones, I believe, are the answer. This is the treatment I am taking, and that thousands of other fortunate women have discovered as well.

Natural Hormone Treatment

Micronized progesterone in transdermal cream, 5–7 mg/kg of body weight per day of therapy.

Estradiol, 0.006–0.009 mg/kg of body weight per day of therapy.

Testosterone, 0.01 mg/kg of body weight per day of therapy. (*Note:* Apply to labia and around the clitoris.)

Continuous administration for two to four months, followed by five-day hiatus.

Testosterone is used less frequently and usually in conjunction with combination therapy. Again, the duration of this treatment is dictated by the patient's needs and the doctor's advice.

GROUP V:
MENOPAUSAL AND POSTMENOPAUSAL
Age: Fifty-five-plus

Symptoms:

Mood swings	*Sleep disorders*
Bloating	*Migraines*
Weight gain	*Hair loss*
Digestive problems	*Hot flashes*
Night sweats	*Loss of sex drive*
Depression and anxiety	*Cardiac disease*
Bone density depletion	

Menstrual Status: Complete cessation

Donna, a fifty-seven-year-old in my practice, told me that she wished her mother, who had osteoporosis, had taken natural hormones. Her mother died at sixty-three from complications of a fractured hip. Donna has been on my natural hormone regimen since she was fifty-four. She's thin, vivacious, healthy, and tells me she feels thirty-five. She certainly looks it.

Sophie is a seventy-eight-year-old retired nurse. She has always taken good care of herself. She had heard about natural hormones years ago but could not convince her gynecologist to look into their availability. She said her gynecologist told her she was too old to start hormones in her seventies. She didn't believe him. Instead, she found a compounding pharmacy and had jars of progesterone cream sent to her. She took a scoop a day and began to feel better (I don't recommend this type of self-dosing; you should always work with your doctor.) She came to me because she thought a more controlled dosing method would work better. It did. She's been with me for four years.

Natural Hormone Treatment

Micronized progesterone in transdermal cream, 5–7 mg/kg of body weight per day of therapy.

Estradiol, 0.006–0.009 mg/kg of body weight per day of therapy.

I've had patients on this regimen for three years, and I have no intention of stopping them in the foreseeable future. Every day, new data are generated on the positive long-term effects of natural hormones. Used in moderation by a knowledgeable physician in conjunction with a reputable pharmacy that specializes in compounding natural hormones, I personally believe patients will successfully use natural hormones indefinitely. I see no reason why I won't use them myself for at least the next fifty years.

Discuss the above guidelines with your doctor to develop a therapeutic program that works best for you.

LONG-TERM USE OF NATURAL HORMONE SUPPLEMENTATION

In References, at the end of this book, you'll find the studies available on the effects of long-term usage of natural hormone supplementation. Because my goal is to bring doctors and patients together on the topic of natural hormones, I have listed scientific studies conventional physicians will respect alongside lay literature accessible to non-medical folks. Scientific studies that evaluate safety and efficacy of natural progesterone and estrogen support our clinical findings. Despite my extensive research, I have not seen literature about negative side effects; absorption in transdermal formulations has been found to be consistently reliable. Natural hormone supplementation (in prescriptive dosing) appears to be the best method of hormone treatment to address symptoms of hormone imbalance without creating negative side effects or any known long-term dangers to the user. Although the number of references is sometimes limited, clinicians who are familiar with natural hormone therapies find their beneficial effects remarkable.

When researching overall hormone replacement therapies, conventional scientific studies provide an array of confusing and contradictory information. The majority of findings published in medical literature are based on data obtained from studies on hormone replacement therapy with synthetic hormones. When you read about the latest results of scientific data on hormone replacement, you enter the world of statistics—a world that specializes in trying to find common denominators for individual needs. Some data assure us of the protection estrogen provides against heart disease and osteoporosis, while other data contradict.

Statistics, however, do not apply to the individual. Statistics refer to population trends and can be manipulated to fit expected results. Many research analysts base their statistics on small groups of patients treated with only synthetic hormones. The results, thus, are often skewed and don't take into consideration the positive impact of natural hormone supplementation. Because the studies often exclusively analyze synthetic hormones, their results can be misleading. To the public, the data can be confusing because we've been indoctrinated into believing that hormones and synthetic preparations are the same thing.

When deciding what type of hormone treatment you choose, I caution you against relying solely on statistics. I also caution you to find out who sponsored the studies you or your doctor are using to make decisions by. Talk to women (and physicians) who have tried both—what better way could there be to gauge whether natural hormones are right for you?

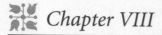 *Chapter VIII*

Clearing Up the Confusion About Medical Testing

*M*edical testing is paramount to good care. Because medicine is truly a fine combination of art and science, diverging opinions on what adequate testing should be can be found in all medical journals, as well as lay sources of information (popular literature, women's journals, TV shows and news, and newspapers). Day in and day out, I'm faced with the same questions from my new patients: "What tests will you use to determine what hormone regimen to choose for me? How will you work to minimize the risks of potential dangers of hormone treatment? How will you measure the effectiveness of treatment?"

To properly answer these questions, we must realize that the issue of testing straddles two worlds. The first is the world of conventional medicine, where all testing is geared toward uncovering disease. This world includes preventive medicine, a branch of conventional medicine that focuses on early diagnosis of disease, not prevention of illness. The second is the world of wellness. That world is caught between conventional medicine and alternative practices. Most people belong in the world of wellness. The average person spends most of his or her life healthy. Illnesses represent minor interruptions in the continuum of health. More than 90 percent of the world's population never see a doctor in their lifetime. In the world of wellness, everyone has one common goal: to prolong the healthy periods and shorten or minimize the interruptions caused by illnesses. This is the world of true prevention, and this is where natural hormones belong. This is a brave new world whose goal is to use the medical information we have about our genetic makeup, environment, and lifestyle to improve our odds for prolonged health and vitality. Wellness is about making women feel better, enjoying life, removing bothersome symptoms of hormone depletion, and ultimately preventing disease.

The easiest way to measure success in the field of natural hormone supplementation is through elimination of symptoms. Thus, symptom relief is the primary goal. The problem is that no medical test can give you this information. Only you, the woman taking the hormone supplementation, can determine how successful your particular program is.

Once we understand that symptom relief is the most important marker of how successful our hormone supplementation treatment is, we can integrate conventional medical testing into our overall surveillance program. We want to stay well, and we want to prevent disease, but we also need to use modern medicine to diagnose early signs of trouble. It's at this point that your conventional doctor becomes invaluable in your care. Once your doctor understands that natural hormones will provide you with symptom relief, and that this is the only way to measure their success in your care, conventional medical surveillance can be useful to you for early diagnosis of disease.

Following is a list of tests currently recommended and performed in conventional medicine as part of routine medical maintenance. Ask your physician to order them to track safety of medication over time, maintain high standards of care, and keep you in the loop of conventional medical progress.

PAP SMEAR

Your gynecologist will not discourage you from having annual or even biannual Pap smears. Pap smears reflect the cellular makeup of a sample taken from the mouth of the uterus, the cervix. The test was developed to diagnose early cervical abnormalities that are easily, safely, and successfully treated. Statistically, the standard profile for women at high risk for getting cervical cancer describes young women in their twenties, of less affluent background, with multiple sexual partners. If you don't qualify under the above categorization, your chances of getting cervical cancer are negligible, and the need for Pap tests more than once a year is questionable. In fact, as of the year 2000, the National Institutes of Health recommends that women with two consecutively normal Pap smears a year apart do not need Pap smears on a yearly basis.

Confer with your gynecologist about the frequency of Pap smears indicated for your particular situation. Keep in mind that the results of a Pap smear do not indicate the effectiveness of hormone therapy.

BLOOD TESTS

When I was a resident at Kings County Hospital, New York, taking 100cc of blood from every patient who was admitted to the hospital was routine. The blood was tested for every diagnosable disease. Today, I believe only those tests whose results will affect the course of treatment should be performed. When you have your examination at the doctor's office, a battery of blood tests is routinely done. I have listed them here, with an overview of their purpose.

General Blood Testing

- Complete blood count (CBC). This test will diagnose anemia as well as revealing your red blood cell count, white blood cell count, and the type of white cells circulating in your blood. This is the most routine of blood tests. Hormone supplementation does not directly affect this test.

- Complete SMAC. This general blood profile reflects general liver, kidney, and metabolic functions; level of hydration of your body; and levels of calcium, sodium, potassium, bicarbonate, and other basic elements found in your blood. Most normal healthy people have normal SMAC results. Minor abnormalities mean little if unrelated to clinical problems.

- Lipid profile. This is a complete lipids count and their breakdown into good versus bad cholesterol, triglycerides, HDL, LDL, VLDL. Estrogen and progesterone depletion is associated with a rise in cholesterol as well as an increase in bad cholesterol (LDL).

- Thyroid panel—TSH, T3, T4, T7. These tests reflect the status of your thyroid gland's function. The incidence of hypothyroidism (low thyroid) increases with age. The ratio of thyroid slowdown between women and men is 5:1—so make sure you have a yearly thyroid function screening test.

The above tests should be performed every year or eighteen months as part of your routine health maintenance program. Abnormalities in the context of clinical problems will enable your doctor to diagnose and treat illness early.

Hormone Blood Testing

Most medical experts agree that following blood hormone levels is not useful in the treatment of symptoms of hormone deficiency. Performing blood hormone level testing is a matter of comfort for both doctors and patients. The frequency of testing should be guided by signs and symptoms that lead the physician to suspect potential illness, not hormone balance in healthy individuals. Tests used to evaluate hormone production and end-organ response (how the ovaries, testes, and adrenal glands function) are as follows:

- Follicle-stimulating hormone (FSH). This is a test of the function of the pituitary gland (master gland). A repeatedly elevated number tells you that your ovaries and adrenals are not making enough estrogen and progesterone. The pituitary gland goes into overdrive, sending desperate signals to your ovaries and adrenals—as well as the corpus luteum—to make more estrogen, progesterone, and testosterone. The only use for this test is to reinforce what you already know when you're in full-blown menopause—you're hormone deficient. All the symptoms you're experiencing just reinforce the blood test. If you're in your thirties or forties, have had breast cancer, and have been placed on tamoxifen, an elevated FSH actually tells you that the tamoxifen has thrown you into menopause. If you're taking fertility pills and your FSH is consistently elevated, you could be experiencing ovarian failure.

- Luteinizing hormone (LH). This is the other hormone produced by the pituitary gland that reflects signs of ovulation. The test is unnecessary for the management of hormone supplementation in older women who are already known to be menopausal. Its only use is in fertility studies. It reflects whether you've ovulated or not. The time of the month when this hormone level is tested is critical for women trying to get pregnant. Another potential use for testing LH level is to correlate it to the night sweats you're experiencing. An interesting theory for the motivator behind night sweats is that the pituitary gland sends pulses of luteinizing hormone (LH) in the middle of the night in an attempt to stimulate the end organs—adrenals and ovaries—to make more estrogen and progesterone. These hormones become depleted in our forties and on; the LH pulses are thus the pituitary's futile attempt to revive the unresponsive end organs.

- Estrogen (estradiol, estriol, estrone). Estrogen is made of three components with varying levels of activity. When we perform the tests to measure how much estrogen is in our blood, we're able to examine the amounts of estrogen circulating freely and the total amount of estrogen in the bloodstream. Most estrogen is actually bound—tied to other molecules (proteins) and receptors on the cell walls—and cannot be measured by our methods of testing. Depending on which fragment of the estrogen molecule is tested (remember that there are three), we learn only the amount of that particular fragment available for measurement. The information this data gives us has no bearing on how much estrogen is available for use to our body. That sounds awfully complicated—and indeed it is. Most physicians working with hormones don't perform these tests, because we aren't sure what to do with the results, or how they correlate with the patient's symptoms. It would be useful, however, to know how much of the hormone taken by a patient receiving supplementation is getting into the bloodstream. It might also help in the evaluation of the best method of administering a hormone—cream versus pills versus capsules.

For example, I prefer working with estradiol; therefore, the type of estrogen I routinely measure in my patients is estradiol. If the level is normal and the patient is feeling good, everything's fine. The picture grows complicated when, for example, the level is high and the patient is feeling good, or the level is low and the patient feels good. If the level is high, I repeat the test in a couple of months. If it's low, I leave it alone. So much for scientific information! Until we have better methods of measuring hormone levels, we're back to the importance of how you feel.

■ Progesterone. Measuring free and total blood progesterone levels is even less important in guiding a physician in the area of hormone supplementation. The most frequent use for progesterone levels is in the field of infertility.

■ Testosterone. Believed to be an exclusively male hormone, testosterone has now become closely associated with female sex drive. I cannot tell you how often women who come to see me about their diminishing interest in sex start the conversation with questions about testosterone. Everyone wants to try it, but at the same time women are afraid of growing whiskers or becoming baritones. Rest assured, no one becomes a man from taking testosterone supplementation under the supervision of a knowledgeable physician. The doses women need to get their libidos back in gear are so much smaller than the doses needed to turn into men that the risks are limited.

Testosterone levels are seldom tested in women. We don't know enough about the normal values, and as with the other hormones, no studies have correlated testosterone levels to symptoms. In men, however, we do measure free- and total-circulating testosterone levels when we supplement them.

Each one of the above tests reflects the level of a given hormone at a stagnant point in time. It's important to remember, however, that the human body is a beautiful dynamic system. By taking a blood test here and there, we are doing a disservice and simplifying an intricate system. Taking a snapshot will never reflect the moving picture. Unless we start measuring hormone levels multiple times a day and week and month, accurate interpretation of the results is impossible. If you have these levels tested once or twice a year, there's absolutely nothing your doctor can determine from the results. The only possible use for these tests would be as part of a poorly constructed attempt to correlate symptoms with hormone levels.

SALIVA TESTING

This test is a new and easy method of determining free hormone levels available for use in the saliva. It's performed by a few mail-order laboratories; data on the usefulness of this test are largely anecdotal. Still, it's cheap, it isn't invasive, and it can be made available to practically anyone. No doctor's order is necessary.

According to its proponents, saliva testing offers a good measurement of the amount of free hormones available for use by the body at a particular point in time. For women who are taking hormone supplementation, a saliva test may be a fairly reliable indicator of the hormones' bioavailability. The problem with the test is the same as with any other test of hormones: It reflects one point in time and offers no overview of the general status of the hormone balance in your body.

TWENTY-FOUR-HOUR URINE TESTING

A rarely used test, the twenty-four-hour urine hormone test has been advocated by Jonathan Wright, MD, one of the original proponents of natural hormone therapy. The test is cumbersome, costly, and difficult to interpret. Unlike the snapshot approach taken by blood testing, twenty-four-hour urine will reflect the quantity of hormones excreted through your kidneys in twenty-four hours. It does not, however, reflect variation of hormone levels with the time of day—an important piece of information when using this test in infertility therapy. Unless the test is performed at short time intervals following or during hormone therapy, its use in menopause is limited.

BONE DENSITY

Bone density studies are important when setting a course for the future. Before taking a bone density test, risk assessment should be the primary mode of screening. If you're small framed and thin and your mother—even if not diagnosed with osteoporosis—was stooped over, you're at high risk.

A baseline bone density test for women over fifty provides information about the thickness of a woman's bones at a critical point when estrogen, which protects us from thinning bones, starts to wane. There are quite a number of bone density tests available, so it's important to know how reliable they are and what type of information they give you.

For a baseline test in people who have no family history of osteoporosis, don't smoke, exercise regularly, and are on a bone-sparing diet, a simple ultrasound of the heel will do. I personally like this test, because it reflects the thickness of a much-stressed bone. Since we're constantly pounding down on our heels, signs of thinning in this bone should lead to more in-depth evaluation of the general status of your skeletal system.

Another popular test—performed right in the doctor's office—measures the thickness of the middle finger bone. I find this test of questionable value, because the bone tested is very small and not necessarily representative of the state of your spine or hip or legs—the areas where osteoporosis does the earliest and most significant damage.

For people with a family history of osteoporosis, poor eating habits, and a history of cancer including chemotherapy, or who are taking tamoxifen or other anti-estrogen medications, the bone density test should be a DEXA scan. This compares the thickness of your hip, femur or forearm, and spine to what's considered normal for your age group and body configuration.

For women at risk who are taking hormones or medications to improve bone density, following bone density levels on a yearly basis is a wise choice.

If your bone density was normal as a baseline and you aren't at risk genetically, are taking natural hormones, are eating well, taking calcium, magnesium, and vitamin D supplements, and exercising regularly, it's unnecessary to repeat your bone density level more often than every two years.

A word of caution about bone density testing. This test

came into vogue when a pharmaceutical company started making medication specifically aimed at "treating" osteoporosis. Free heel or finger testing is often sponsored by the drug manufacturers; the goal may be to find as many women as possible with thinning bones to place on medications. To date—almost five years since the medication has come to market—there are no data to support the medication's beneficial results in the reversal or prevention of osteoporosis. Diet, exercise, and natural hormone supplementation present a much more benign and promising way to protect ourselves from osteoporosis.

CARDIAC STRESS TESTING

Women over the age of forty whose hormones are beginning to deplete rapidly catch up with men in incidence of heart disease. Women over fifty have the same incidence of heart disease as men. Heart disease is the number one killer of older women. Until ten years ago, the medical profession seemed totally unaware of this important public health issue—but the picture, fortunately, is changing. Cardiac stress testing is now considered a good method to diagnose heart disease long before a woman has a heart attack, as her risk factors increase with age.

The most commonly used stress test is the sesta MIBI—a treadmill test in which the patient receives a radioactive injection, which helps visualize the blood vessels of the heart. The test is safe and quite reliable; it has been a staple for testing men (AKA thallium test) for the past fifteen years. A positive or abnormal test is usually followed by angiography, also known as coronary arteriography. The angiogram is a more invasive test, but it's not just a diagnostic test. If it's abnormal, it becomes a therapeutic test: An angioplasty—cleaning out the clogged blood vessels—is often performed at the same time.

The newest test for screening heart problems is the ultrafast CT scan—EBCT. It's a noninvasive test. A CT scan is performed that identifies areas of calcification in the coronary artery system. If the test is positive, the same route as for a regular stress test is followed.

MAMMOGRAPHY

Mammography is a radiologic test used to diagnose breast cancer. It's not a preventive measure. Mammography diagnoses breast cancer once it is there. It doesn't protect us from getting breast cancer, and it doesn't prevent breast cancer from growing. I can't tell you how many patients, myself included, go through weeks if not months of sheer panic before going to have their annual mammograms, for fear of a positive reading. The more exposed we are to the importance of having yearly mammograms, the more stressed out and paranoid we become about the risk for breast cancer.

The tissue that makes up our breasts is the most radiosensitive tissue in the body. Every time we have a mammogram, we're exposing it to radiation in the name of protection. If you ask the radiologists, they'll tell you not to worry; the dosage of radiation is very low. As a doctor, however, I feel uncomfortable that with each passing year, we are ordering more mammograms and promote the importance of this test without addressing the dangers of radiation to the very breasts we're trying to protect.

When I have this conversation about my ambivalence toward the test with my patients, we quickly discover that we're all confused. We don't want to miss the cancer, but we also don't want to stimulate its potential growth by unnecessary exposure to radiation. Regardless, I do have to give direction to the patients I see every day—not to mention figuring out what to do myself.

I have finally achieved a level of comfort with the following compromise.

I suggest a baseline mammogram in all my patients between the ages of thirty-five and forty. Following that, I teach patients self-examination as the most important method of early detection. I recommend mammograms every one to three years, on an individual basis depending on family history, environmental risk factors (diet, smoking, profession), medications (Premarin, tamoxifen, birth control pills), and the presence of persistent lumps.

When I find myself experiencing difficulty making a decision, I use ultrasound to help. Breast ultrasound helps distinguish between solid and hollow masses in the breast. A hollow cyst is less likely to be cancerous than a solid one. When I reach the point where no other doctor—meaning radiologist—will commit, I opt for a biopsy of the exact area in question. Stereotactic biopsies (fine needle aspirations under fluoroscopic guidance) are the only type of biopsy you should allow. The abnormality is identified in the radiology suite by a radiologist; then, under direct visualization, a fine wire is threaded into the area in question for the surgeon to extract.

PELVIC ULTRASOUND: THE BEST WAY TO FOLLOW THE EFFECTS OF HORMONE TREATMENT

I am amazed how little this incredibly valuable test is being used. Most gynecologists have easy access to ultrasound machines, and most radiologic facilities have more than one type of ultrasound machine. Yet unless they're pregnant or are being studied for infertility, few women undergo this test as part of routine health maintenance programs.

Without a doubt, in my opinion every woman on hormone supplementation—whether natural or synthetic—should have annual pelvic ultrasounds. It's an inexpensive test—but the information derived from it is priceless. It allows your physician to determine the thickness of the lining of your uterus and visualize the shape and configuration of your ovaries. This method of follow-up is important, because hormone supplementation directly affects both your uterus and ovaries. The thickness of the uterine lining is directly affected by both estrogen and progesterone. The more estrogen, the thicker the lining; the more progesterone, the thinner. Good balance between the two translates into normal thickness. In addition, the ovaries are constantly under the direct effect of hormones.

Ultrasound is the test that provides the best basic information necessary to evaluate hormone therapy of any kind.

Ovarian Cysts and the Use of Ultrasound

When a twenty-two-year-old goes to a doctor with pain in her lower abdomen, the doctor thinks: *ovarian cyst*. There are more ultrasounds of the pelvis ordered on young women with bellyaches than probably any other test. Why are we so attuned to ovarian cysts in our twenties—but then forget about them as we age?

Ovarian cysts are not necessarily abnormal. They're common, and their presence isn't automatically a warning sign of potential disease nor an indication for surgical intervention. In chapter 2, I talked about the corpus luteum. When we ovulate, the egg is pushed out of the ovary. At the site on the ovary from which the egg was pushed out, a cyst sometimes develops. This cyst may be hollow or filled with fluid or tissues; it grows or shrinks under the influence of circulating hormones. Occasionally, it becomes large enough to cause discomfort. Rarely, it ruptures and causes severe pain. Most commonly, the cyst disappears before the beginning of the next period. When we take hormones of any type (starting with birth control pills), the ovaries often react by forming cysts. Ultrasound is the best way to follow the evolution of these cysts. The rare times when cysts necessitate surgical intervention is when they become large and painful or when they're diagnosed as tumors (most often benign).

Why Use Ultrasound in Older Women?

When hormone therapy is administered, the ovary is stimulated and, sometimes, cysts grow. They are most often benign, and monitoring them with periodic ultrasounds is an appropriate and safe approach.

You should also know that the late diagnosis of ovarian cancer in women over forty can have deadly effects. The easiest way to diagnose ovarian cancer early is to perform routine ultrasounds of women at high risk.

CAT SCANNING AND MRI

If an ultrasound reveals abnormalities, the next step is obtaining a CAT scan and/or MRI. These are highly sophisticated tests and need not be used routinely. Conventional medicine has developed logical and safe sequential approaches to diagnosing illness; let your physician guide you. Our goal is to keep you healthy and prevent illness. CAT scanning and MRIs have little place in the evaluation of healthy people.

TESTING REGIMEN FOR
HORMONE SOLUTION PATIENTS

Balancing natural hormone supplementation should be based on symptom relief. We do not yet have accurate enough guidelines in blood testing to correlate blood levels to hormone balance; ultrasound is the only test that will show the effects of hormones. Still, this doesn't mean you should forgo testing altogether. Work with your doctor to find the tests that reflect your symptom status and create a blend of subjective and objective guidelines to best suit your individual needs.

To deal with the conflicting information and provide the patients in my practice with safety and good follow-up, I advise the following testing regimen:

- A baseline mammogram at age thirty-five to forty for women with no family history of cancer or other risk factors.

- A baseline CBC, SMAC, hormone, thyroid, lipid blood test at the initial visit, and then follow-up based on individual needs and symptoms on a biyearly or yearly basis.

- A stress test for all women over fifty.

- A Pap smear yearly for menstruating women, and every other year for women who have stopped their menses.

- A baseline bone density test for women over forty; repeat at yearly intervals if the family history suggests high risk for osteoporosis or the woman is on chemotherapy or anti-estrogen medication.

- An ultrasound of the pelvis at the initial evaluation, and yearly for all patients on hormone supplementation.

- A baseline colonoscopy for women fifty and above with no family history of colon cancer.

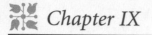

Chapter IX

Synthetic Hormones and Cancer

Hormones are very powerful molecules. Understanding their role in our lives and the impact they have on everything we do gives me pause. Before we discuss whether synthetic hormones have been associated with cancer, a few critical concepts must be understood.

Let's say you drive to work every day, and always take the same route. You pass the same houses, the same trees, the same scenery every day for years. You think you know the road like the back of your hand. Then suddenly one day you notice a yellow house on your right. It's not new, it's always been there; you just haven't noticed it before.

Has this ever happened to you?

It's a common occurrence, and it just reinforces that we are all human; our brain, no matter how intelligent and perceptive, can take in only a limited amount of information at any given time. And then randomly, one day, the brain opens up and allows a little more information to penetrate the conscious mind.

That's exactly what happened to me with regard to natural versus synthetic hormones. As a conventional physician, I believed that estrogen—the hormone our body makes—and synthetic estrogen substitutes were similar enough to be interchangeable. This belief was founded in my education. My medical school training led me to believe that estrogen replacement in menopause consisted exclusively of synthetic hormones. Although scientific data questioning the safety and the efficacy of synthetic hormone replacement abound in medical literature, natural hormones were not an option. It took almost a decade of private practice to bring me to the point where my mind opened up, understood, and welcomed the difference between natural and synthetic hormones.

Let's spend a little time understanding the significance of the difference.

SYNTHETIC HORMONES

Estrogen

Estrogen is a natural hormone made by the ovaries and adrenals of every human—indeed, every mammal—in the world. It defines certain critical female characteristics and has a wide array of effects. Until the mid-1960s, the main thing doctors knew about estrogen was its effect and importance in the human body in its natural form. In 1966, Robert Wilson, a physician, wrote a book called *Feminine Forever.* The book equated estrogen with youth. Supported by a large pharmaceutical company that had received a patent on the synthetic estrogen Premarin, the book was an immense success. It appealed to women's desire to stay young and attractive as well as free of menopausal symptoms.

This success meant more than just skyrocketing sales for the book—and for Premarin; it was also a turning point. As a result of this successful marketing campaign, Americans started to identify estrogen with Premarin. Thus, the difference between natural estrogen made by our bodies and synthetic estrogen was blurred in the minds of the public—and the medical profession as well.

While this situation created a boon for the Premarin

industry, it was not clear that it always helped women feel better. Even those physicians and women who felt that Premarin was not a complete panacea had few readily available alternatives. Without the help of conventional doctors (many of whom were unfamiliar with them), and without mainstream support, natural hormones entered the market through the back door. And as it gradually became apparent that natural hormones produce beneficial clinical results, increasing numbers of physicians engaged in the battle to separate the two—estrogen from Premarin!

When I talk about estrogen, I am only referring to the hormone naturally made by our body, not the synthetic substitutes made in laboratories. This estrogen defines us as women: It makes our breasts grow, it brings on our periods, it makes the lining of the uterus grow, it makes us ovulate, it prepares us for and supports pregnancy as well as the growth of the fetus inside the womb. It also helps protect us from heart disease, makes our bones strong, and keeps our metabolism running in high gear. Mother Nature ensures the perpetuation of the human species by revving up our body's hormone production. When we're young, our body manufactures large quantities of estrogen in order to fulfill our calling. High levels of estrogen bathe our organs during pregnancy. These high levels don't make us sick—as a matter of fact, they make us glow and keep us healthy. With this knowledge in mind, synthetic estrogen was developed. No pharmaceutical company would have created an estrogenlike substance (trying to duplicate the effects of the natural molecule) if estrogen itself had been perceived as dangerous.

When Robert Wilson's book was published in 1966, estrogen, along with its synthetic version, Premarin, made its grand entrance as the sole hormone of importance in women's well-being. While every endocrinology textbook then and now stresses the equal importance of progesterone in the maintenance of normal hormone balance in women, progesterone was not brought to the market when Premarin emerged. The women who took Premarin in the 1960s were limited in numbers, and few seemed to register complaints with their doctors.

A key point to remember was that menopause was not an openly discussed topic in those days. A woman's role was still limited to the home, to having and raising children; women were not a major presence in the marketplace. The women's movement was just beginning, and its leaders were more concerned with birth control than menopause. Some women didn't even know menopause existed. Our mothers never talked about it. I never even knew my mother went through menopause—and I was a doctor! I remember once hearing about a distant great-aunt who went crazy in midlife and ended up in a mental institution, but no connection was ever made between mental or physical problems and menopause. Menopause was a deep, dark secret hidden in the back of women's closets. So without public demand, pharmaceutical companies had no motivation to look any further into the area of female hormones. Premarin remained the best-known option.

By the 1970s, things started to change. Studies began to link Premarin therapy to an increased incidence in uterine cancer. At the same time, studies on birth control pills (which also contained high doses of synthetic estrogen) started to connect their use to increased incidence of blood clots in the legs and lungs. This prompted a flurry of studies searching for alternatives. Although low-dose estrogen birth control pills did start to arrive on the market, the basic makeup of birth control pills has remained the same to this day—synthetic hormones.

At the time, I was in medical school, and I distinctly

remember seeing patients experiencing the side effects of synthetic estrogens described in the scientific articles I was reading. In the clinics of Kings County Hospital, I saw women with swollen breasts, heavy irregular periods, ovarian cysts, phlebitis, and pulmonary embolisms. I believed that many of these were the living and breathing connections to the effects of synthetic estrogens reported in the medical literature. With all good intentions, we had started these patients on synthetic hormones—and now we were faced with problems we'd never expected. We hadn't considered possible side effects such as toxicity to sex organs overstimulated by synthetic high-dose estrogen replacement. And why would we? Pharmaceuticals and medicine were still on their honeymoon.

But like most honeymoons, this one ended. In many respects, it created a long-lasting marriage; still, many unanswered questions started to arise. Slowly but surely, data on significant side effects of synthetic hormones appeared in the medical and lay literature. Women started to react. Many stopped taking Premarin, and many stopped taking birth control pills. Unfortunately, a lot of women continued with these medications. Some were afraid to disobey their doctors. Many were scared even to tell their doctors of problems they were having with the medications, and some just ignored the side effects and simply accepted them as part of their lives.

Others, with the guidance of a few then-revolutionary physicians, turned to the forgotten hormone—progesterone—for help with hormone balance and protection from estrogen dominance and its now-well-documented dangers.

Progesterone

At this time, there was still no mass-produced progesterone on the market—but pharmaceutical companies recognized the demand for it. Still, just as with estrogen, the most lucrative way to market progesterone is to make a synthetic substance and secure a patent. Enter progestin. Progestin as in Provera, Prempro, and Premphase became the solution to the problems Premarin alone could not solve. But progestin is not progesterone—and that's another source of confusion to the public.

With the arrival of synthetic progesterone, both doctors and patients had lost the battle to separate synthetic from natural hormones. The market was flooded with the two synthetic preparations; the natural hormone option did not even appear to exist.

All of the above are hormone impostors, in the sense that they're synthetically manufactured to fool our bodies into believing that we're getting the hormones we need. But unfortunately, synthetic hormones cannot completely fool our bodies, and ultimately we may pay a high price for using them. Let's go back to the synthetic hormones known as progestins. In our bodies, they accomplish two goals, neither of which we really need for healthy function:

1. They compete with whatever hormones our bodies are producing by taking up receptor sites.

2. They create new receptors for their foreign molecules on our cells. This confuses the cells and stimulates a defensive immune response.

When synthetic hormones became popular in the mid-1960s, their long-term effects could not be anticipated, but many signs of their incompatibility with the human body were immediately recognizable. Unfortunately, many women taking them either ignored their side effects or went off the medications. Thus important information about the medications' shortcomings were rarely shared with their doctors.

I remember distinctly feeling very sick the first month I took birth control pills at the age of nineteen. I was placed on them because I had severe menstrual cramps. My doctor told me to bear with it because they would eliminate my cramps; as an added bonus, I would be protected from getting pregnant. I was not sexually active. All I had was bad cramps. Within three weeks I had migraines, became bloated and moody, and felt like I was living in another person's body. I called my doctor and asked if my new symptoms could have anything to do with the birth control pills. He told me it was very unlikely. I stopped taking the pills after two months and I never went back to that doctor. I also never called him to tell him why. He may still be prescribing those birth control pills and thinking the patients are taking them, even if they aren't. I know now that I should have told him; I might have helped both him and other women.

When I started practicing medicine, I listened to this same story from many of my healthy young patients who were taking birth control pills. When they complained of headaches, I gave them medication; when they became bloated, I gave them some more medication. It took many years for me to realize that there may be a connection between the medication and the problems. Today, if a young woman has side effects from birth control pills, I advise her to discontinue the pills and use other methods of contraception. I've found that if one of my patients reacts with significant side effects to one type of birth control pill, her chances of better tolerating another are minimal. I don't like to suggest any synthetic hormones for birth control any longer. The full story on potential long-term effects of birth control pills on fertility, cancer, and early induction of menopause has not been investigated. While data on the use of natural hormones for birth control are slowly percolating, the results thus far appear promising. In my practice, I prescribe natural hormones for women over forty with good results. Although I often prescribe natural hormones along with diaphragms or IUDs, my patients are happy and virtually free of side effects.

Let's go back and take a closer look at the use of synthetic estrogens beyond childbearing age. When placed in the human body, synthetic estrogen acts like estrogen in one important respect: It makes breast and endometrial tissue grow. Its significant difference from human estrogen is that it's synthetic and thus a foreign substance to our bodies. Remember, Premarin contains equinil. Equinil, the horse-specific estrogen, is a molecule foreign to our bodies. When it attaches to our cellular receptors, our immune system tries to fight it off. The normal bodily means of defending itself from foreign molecules (horse protein in this case) is to insulate them by building walls around them or creating a systemic immune response. This could even be something as serious as a tumor or an abscess; allergies, migraines, or rashes. On a cellular level, the reaction is even more dramatic. A cover article in *Time* magazine in 1995 called "The Estrogen Dilemma" raised questions about the use of estrogen. Two scientific studies—published in 1998 and 1999 in *Chemical Research in Toxicology* and *Proceedings of the Society for Biological Medicine*—proved that once broken down in our bodies, equilin becomes toxic to the very DNA that keeps us healthy or makes us sick. For me and my practice, the information introduced and the questions raised were sufficient to provide the final nail in the coffin of synthetic estrogen. I would never prescribe them again. The risk was too high, the rewards too low. Suddenly, all the side effects, the questions, and the doubts I had about synthetic estrogens became too overwhelming for me to continue prescribing them.

ENDOMETRIAL/UTERINE CANCER

In the average woman, estrogen causes the lining of the uterus to grow. Progesterone is the only way the body has to prevent unchecked growth stimulated by estrogen. Progesterone balances estrogen by turning off the cell-growth mechanism—it makes cells stop growing. Thus, it prevents overgrowth of the uterine lining (also known as the endometrium). The incidence of uterine cancer seemed to rise with the treatment of menopausal symptoms with unopposed synthetic estrogens.

Between the 1960s when Premarin came to the market and the 1970s when the data on endometrial cancer started to appear in the medical literature, more and more women were treated with Premarin alone without the invaluable balancing effect of progesterone. The Endometrial Cancer Cooperative Group first established the probable relationship between estrogen replacement and the risk of endometrial cancer. Its studies showed that the menopausal women who took synthetic estrogen for one to five years experienced a threefold increase in incidence of uterine cancer. Those who took synthetic estrogen for ten years had a tenfold increase. Lifetime use of synthetic estrogen potentially increased a woman's chance of getting uterine cancer to one in ten.

Although when I went through my medical training in the mid- to late 1970s, unopposed synthetic estrogen therapy for menopausal symptoms began to be questioned, all too many women were still being treated with synthetic estrogens without balancing them with any type of progesterone. I remember being taught that although the incidence of deaths from uterine cancer had increased two- to threefold in the years since Premarin, uterine cancer was a low-grade cancer. A 1993 study by the Endometrial Cancer Collaborative Group published in *Unresolved Issues* found that uterine cancer associated with treatment with Premarin had a 90 percent cure rate, as compared to uterine cancer in general, with a cure rate of only 70 to 75 percent. This may sound good to a statistician, but it still troubled me. I went into medicine to take care of patients, not statistics. My professors of obstetrics and gynecology were quick to point out that as soon as we figured out the need to balance estrogen (synthetic estrogen) with progestin (synthetic progesterone), the risk of developing uterine cancer was practically eliminated. It was just common sense. Unfortunately, they were right with respect to the cancer risk, but I became concerned that in practice we weren't balancing with progesterone, we were trying to balance with yet another synthetic substance.

As a young doctor desperately wanting to help my patients and believing in the system that educated me, I took the information to heart and started menopausal patients I saw on the new combination drugs: Prempro, Premphase, or cycled Premarin and Provera. But as a measure of caution, I did make sure these women were given uterine ultrasounds on a twice-a-year basis. For me, a young resident in 1977, that seemed to work. Premarin took away the hot flashes; Provera made women feel younger because they continued to have periods. I figured that that was good. I was in my twenties, and I didn't realize that fifty-five-year-olds don't normally have periods.

Then in 1994, a landmark study was published in the *American Journal of Obstetrics and Gynecology* by J. D.

Woodruff and J. H. Pickar: "Incidence of Endometrial Hyperplasia in Postmenopausal Women Taking Conjugated Estrogens (Synthetic) with Medroxyprogesterone Acetate or Conjugated Estrogens Alone." This article addressed an extensive study on the effects on the uterine lining of four different regimens of combinations of synthetic estrogen and progestin and synthetic estrogen alone. The duration of the study was one year; it involved approximately a thousand women. The results established that treating women with synthetic estrogen alone could drastically increase the risk of endometrial disease, while combinations of synthetic estrogen with synthetic progesterone helped reduce the risk.

Since that time, other studies have validated the findings described in the Woodruff study. While factually the information gathered from these studies is accurate—unopposed estrogen therapy can increase the risk of uterine cancer—no natural hormone solution was offered. All these studies address only the use of synthetic hormones.

To provide a realistic picture of the effects of hormone therapy, treatment with combinations of natural estrogens and progesterones must also be evaluated. Unfortunately, they haven't been adequately studied. Since the studies are costly, and synthetic hormones are profitably manufactured by large commercial pharmaceutical companies, there's more incentive to investigate synthetic substances. The situation leaves a very important question unanswered: Is the increased rate of endometrial cancer associated with estrogen in general or with synthetic estrogen in particular? Common sense suggests to me that synthetic substances could be potentially harmful simply because they're a foreign substance; acquiring comparable therapeutic benefits from a natural substance seems to be a better option.

Still, these studies, incomplete as they were, did appear to provide some comfort to us doctors. Prolonged use of unopposed estrogen may cause uterine cancer, while the combination of synthetic estrogen and progestin eliminates some of this risk. So doctors continued to write prescriptions for synthetic hormones.

Let's not forget another piece of information that the research revealed: Estrogen, the hormone made by our body, has practically no known connection with endometrial cancer. We can deduce this from the fact that the average woman who has never taken hormone replacements rarely, if ever, gets endometrial cancer. According to a 1998 article in the *American Journal of Obstetrics and Gynecology*, it occurs in less than one in a thousand women each year. (Note that this number is based only on information obtained from women who have pelvic examinations—and less than 10 percent of women do.) When evaluating the data, let's note that natural hormones are similar to our own, are milder in their effect than synthetics, and allow flexible dosing.

OVARIAN CANCER

On March 21, 2001, the *Journal of the American Medical Association* reported on a fifteen-year study conducted by the American Cancer Society. This study correlated that women who had taken estrogen replacement for more than ten years between 1982 and 1996 had double the normal risk of dying from ovarian cancer.

Within forty-eight hours of its publication, the data was reviewed by academic medical centers and reported in the media and questions were raised about its statistical significance.

LouAnn died of ovarian cancer at forty-six in 1996. She was single, had no children, and had been taking Prempro for fifteen years because of a family history of osteoporosis and heart disease. When she became my patient, she had already been diagnosed with ovarian cancer and had undergone surgery and chemotherapy. They didn't work. I provided more hospice care for her than medical care. Sadly, I watched her wither away and die without much more than kindness to offer.

After the publication of the ovarian cancer study in 2001, I couldn't help but wonder about LouAnn. Yes, she was at higher risk of getting ovarian cancer because she had no children. But for me, LouAnn's long-term use of Prempro emphasized the need for further studies so that any questions could be put to rest for both patients and doctors.

BREAST CANCER

Although 80 percent of women who get breast cancer have no identifiable common risk factors, contributory factors, genetic and environmental, must be seriously taken into consideration. Breast cancer is a hormone-dependent cancer. Continuous exposure to high levels of unopposed estrogens can increase a woman's chances of getting breast cancer. We may be exposed to too much estrogen when it's out of balance with progesterone; when we're exposed to chemicals, phytoestrogens, and/or radiation; or when we're receiving it in the form of synthetic estrogen replacement therapy.

In 1990, an article titled "The Endocrinology of Breast Cancer" published in *Cancer* established a connection between unopposed estrogen and the development of breast cancer. Since then, studies on synthetic estrogens have only increased the panic women experience living in constant fear of breast cancer. Even though breast cancer is not the number one killer of women, its association with hormone replacement therapy has become the main deterrent to the use of HRT. Unfortunately, the fact that natural progesterone and estrogens may help minimize the risk of breast cancer has been overshadowed by the negative publicity received by their synthetic counterparts.

The *Journal of the American Medical Association* (1977), *Cancer Research* (1973), and *Lancet* (1980)—all reputable and highly respected medical journals—published many articles on the beneficial anticancer effects offered by estriol (natural estrogen). Unfortunately, no large-scale follow-up studies have been undertaken pursuing the benefits of natural hormones since these initial articles appeared more than twenty years ago. The obvious reason: Without sponsorship by pharmaceutical companies, there's little incentive to study them further.

What causes breast cancer? We have no definitive answers, but some risk factors can be highlighted:

- Racial differences and country of residence.
  Caucasian Americans over the age of forty-five are most likely to be diagnosed with breast cancer. This could be purely a function of statistics. Aging American women of middle to higher socioeconomic levels have more mammograms, have more regular checkups, and are targeted by the media for all types of breast cancer awareness activities. In African American women, breast cancer is rarer, with a poorer prognosis and with earlier peak age of incidence. Statistically, the types of breast cancer that African American women often develop are highly virulent and occur in younger women. Research on breast cancer in African American women is comparatively

nonexistent. Asian women are considered the gold standard. They have a very low incidence of breast cancer, and our scientists are in constant debate over the reasons why. Genetics are an obvious factor, but proponents of the miracle of soy have claimed its omnipresence in their diet to be a factor. To date, the jury is out, and research must be directed at the women with high incidence of cancer and their protection.

■ Family history of breast cancer. BRCA (breast cancer) 1 and 2 genes account for 80 percent of inherited cancer cases. Other genes including H-ras, p53 account for other genetically inherited breast cancers. It is important to note that more than 40 percent of women with any of these genetic mutations do not get cancer by the age of seventy. BRCA genes, in the rare instances they are expressed, are associated with breast, ovarian, and colon cancer in women, and prostate and colon cancer in men. Jews of Eastern European origin carry these genes at a 2.3 percent rate. The population at large has less than a 0.003 percent chance of carrying these genes. An Internet group called FORCE provides important communication and support for women carrying these genes.

■ Personal history of breast cancer. Women who have had breast cancer have a fivefold chance of getting breast cancer again in the opposite breast or the same breast. Having a history of breast biopsies also increases the incidence of breast cancer. Scar tissue is formed at the site of the biopsy; the risk of developing cancer in scar tissue has been under investigation by surgical researchers for years. Blind biopsies used to be the standard means to evaluate fibrocystic breasts. Although no definitive connection has been made between fibrocystic breasts and cancer, to this day it's not unusual to hear about doctors just doing a needle biopsy in the office, to quickly get some fluid out and diagnose the content of a breast mass. In my opinion, no woman should allow a doctor to blindly perform an aspiration biopsy. I believe that the only acceptable method of surgically evaluating breast masses is the stereotactic biopsy procedure (see chapter 8).

■ Environmental factors. Chemicals are part of our lives. Exposure to insecticides, other chemicals and synthetic hormones fed to our farm animals, and high-electricity lines in our backyards cannot be ignored as possible factors that contribute to clusters of breast cancer outbreaks.

■ High-animal-fat diets. Women of Western European and American descents—areas where high intake of animal fat is common—can be at higher risk. These women produce more estrogen than women whose diet is mostly vegetables and grains. The statistical difference in incidence of breast cancer is significant—and women of Western European and American descents seem to be at even higher risk if, in addition, we place them on synthetic estrogens and progestins. But to date, there is no method of precisely measuring how each of these factors contributes to the risk.

My approach is to encourage these women to switch to a high-fiber, low-animal-fat diet; to quit smoking; and to supplement with low-dose natural estradiol and micronized progesterone.

John Lee, MD, and the Estrogen Window Hypothesis on Breast Cancer

*A*n interesting and quite logical theory on the development of breast cancer is called the Estrogen Window Hypothesis and has been endorsed by Dr. John Lee, a proponent of natural progesterone therapy. According to this theory, breast cancer often starts during the ten to fifteen years before menopause. It is during this period of time that estrogen is dominant in our bloodstream. As you recall from chapter 1, the quality and quantity of progesterone we make both decrease with age. Hence we live in an estrogen-dominated environment for many years before menopause. According to Dr. Lee, it is during this time that, unchecked by progesterone, breast tissue

DESIGNER ESTROGENS/SERMS

Closely related to the topic of breast cancer is the use of designer estrogens or anti-estrogen drugs. SERMs—selective estrogen receptor modulators—are a new group of drugs. SERMs compete with human estrogen for specific sites on cell receptors. They're synthetic and designed to replace estrogen in certain tissues. They bind to estrogen alpha and estrogen beta receptors and together form a complex structure with divergent effects on human organs.

On uterus and bones, the complex has estrogenlike effects, but on breast tissue it has an anti-estrogen effect. The reason SERMs were developed was to counteract the negative effects of Premarin. SERMs were supposed to pro-

cells keep growing under the stimulation provided by our own internally manufactured estrogen. Considering the average doubling time for breast cancer cells at three to six months, we have eight to ten years to reach a tumor large enough to be diagnosable (by mammogram or palpation).

According to Dr. Lee, if we start supplementing women with micronized progesterone during those eight to ten years of leeway, we might just help save many women from breast cancer. What's the downside of micronized progesterone supplementation? In my view, there are no known serious side effects to date. And that's with more than twenty years of usage.

For more on the Estrogen Window Hypothesis of the etiology of breast cancer, read *Lancet* 1 (1980), pages 700–701.

tect women from increased risk of breast cancer and endometrial cancer.

The two most commonly used SERMs are raloxifene (trade name Evista) and tamoxifen (trade name Nolvadex). A special report published in March 2001 in the journal *Postgraduate Medicine* through a grant by Merck and Company provides an overview of "The Effects of SERMs on Women's Health." Below are some of the specific issues that were raised about the overall effectiveness of the commonly used SERMs:

- While raloxifene has modest positive effects on cardiovascular risk factors, its use is associated with an increased incidence of thromboembolism.

- Phytoestrogens may be less thrombogenic than the currently used formulations of estrogens and synthetic SERMs.

- Cardio protective effect was not confirmed in a recent randomized, placebo-controlled clinical trial.

- The effects of SERMs on brain function are difficult to predict. Regrettably, the number and quality of preclinical and clinical studies conducted thus far to ascertain whether such designer estrogens as tamoxifen and raloxifene have adverse effects on the brain have been inadequate.

Tamoxifen

The "National Surgical Adjuvant Breast and Bowel P-1" trial regarding tamoxifen therapy for breast cancer concluded that:

- Tamoxifen significantly decreased the relative risk of breast cancer—by 49 percent.

- Follow-up on tamoxifen's impact on overall mortality was not available. The authors of the study strongly recommended it be made available.

- Trial results do not apply to the population at large.

- Tamoxifen was not recommended for the prevention of osteoporosis. Women over the age of fifty—who are most likely to be affected by breast cancer—had more adverse effects.

- The benefits did not outweigh the adverse effects.

And yet ten million women are on tamoxifen.

Tamoxifen is prescribed for a minimum of five years in women who have had breast cancer. It's prescribed prophylactically as well. This treatment is based on the results of a National Cancer Institute study that has been questioned repeatedly by English and Italian scientists in articles published in medical journals, including *Lancet.*

In my opinion, this drug should not be used on women with breast cancer or as an option for hormone replacement. Nor should it be used to prevent breast cancer in women at risk. Tamoxifen has been connected to a 2.5 to 7.5 increase in the incidence of uterine cancer. The types of uterine cancers associated with tamoxifen are more aggressive than any other uterine cancer. Tamoxifen has also been associated with increased incidence of blood clots, thrombophlebitis, and pulmonary emboli. It can induce early menopause and its attendant symptoms. Women on tamoxifen may gain weight and/or develop severe night sweats, hot flashes, thinning bones, and heart disease.

As more negative data appear in the literature on tamoxifen, estrogen and progesterone are being reintroduced into the formula for women who have had breast cancer. Once considered taboo, placing women on hormones after breast cancer now appears to be safe and may even help to prevent the cancer's recurrence. Proponents of natural hormones have been saying this for years and often successfully treating women with natural hormones without recurrences or untoward symptoms.

Raloxifene

Raloxifene is another new designer drug with far-reaching medical implications. Its chemical makeup is very similar to tamoxifen's.

Raloxifene was initially developed to treat breast cancer as well. During its clinical trials, it failed to produce the expected therapeutic response in women who had tamoxifen-resistant breast cancer, and it was redirected for use in the treatment of osteoporosis. A study by Delmas and Ettinger concluded that raloxifene was effective in both prevention and treatment of postmenopausal osteoporosis, and the FDA approved its use for these indications. Another role for raloxifene was found in its decrease of LDL cholesterol levels. This prompted a study still in progress—"Raloxifene Use for the Heart (RUTH)"—whose results will be available in 2007. Another study, "Multiple Outcomes of Raloxifene Evaluation (MORE)," provided the following results:

- Raloxifene significantly decreased the relative risk of breast cancer—by 76 percent—in the population studied.

- Raloxifene increased the risk of deep vein thrombosis, pulmonary embolism, and retinal vein thrombosis 3:1.

- Performance on cognitive function tests was not improved.

- LDL cholesterol was decreased, but HDL (good cholesterol) was not increased.

- Bone mineral density was increased, but only minimally.

Side effects may include hot flashes, night sweats, and/or bloating. So far, raloxifene has proven to be of little help for treating hot flashes, improving good cholesterol, or preventing heart disease or Alzheimer's.

Toremifene and Droloxifene

Structurally related to tamoxifen, these are the newest SERMs to hit the market. Their use and the data about them are limited at this time.

All the studies that connect the use of estrogen to cancer refer to the usage of synthetic estrogens. Within that framework, the only statistically significant connection between synthetic estrogens and cancer is between the use of unopposed synthetic estrogens and uterine cancer. Reassuring information comes to us from studies revealing that the combination of even synthetic estrogens with synthetic progesterones (progestins) provides some protection from uterine cancer. Based on the data presently available in the medical literature, I strongly believe that it can be inferred that natural hormones are needed to help minimize the risks of unopposed estrogen as well as of genetic and environmental factors linked to reproductive cancers. As the public understanding of and demand for natural hormones rises, clinical evaluation started in the 1970s and 1980s should resume and must be pursued. This should increase physicians' awareness and use of natural hormones—not only in the treatment of symptoms of hormone deficiency, but also in potentially helping to minimize the risks of cancer.

Chapter X

Diet, Exercise, and Lifestyle

We waste an enormous amount of time trying to fit into a mold created by the media through the women featured on magazine covers, in ads, and in the movies. As a result, we're constantly in search of the magic pill, the magic food, the magic supplement to help us stay thin and look young forever. There is no such thing as one magic solution. Human beings are so complex and so unique that simplistic answers just don't exist. No magic wand will make us stay young forever. Only good genetics and a well-balanced body and mind will keep us in good health. At this point, we know that reaching the ideal balance is directly tied to our hormones. With the aid of natural hormones, we can achieve optimum hormone balance and make life better at any age. But proper hormone balance isn't enough. As we go through life, we cannot overlook the significant contributions of diet, exercise, and lifestyle.

A couple of years ago, I had no trouble identifying my patients' age. Today, as I work exclusively with hormones and rejuvenation, I must admit that I'm often surprised by the youthful appearance and thinking of my patients. Sixty-five-year-olds now look forty more often than not. Yes, they're taking natural hormones, but they also invariably follow a highly successful diet, exercise, and lifestyle program.

All success stories have one thing in common—they feature women who have achieved balance in their lives. A little change in every aspect of our lives brings about a logarithmic improvement in the quality of our lives as a whole.

I don't believe that people will or should follow extreme programs. They don't work. What works is a little change at a time, giving yourself permission not to abide by the rules all the time, and learning to be accepting of yourself even if you don't look like the women on the magazine covers.

DIET

Nothing is more obvious than the fact that we are what we eat. Americans are fatter than ever these days because we eat fast food, chow down while in the car, grab a bite between meetings, and often don't pay attention to the details of our diets.

My motto is, "Junk in, junk out." Based on this simple concept, I believe that if you put into your body highly synthetic processed junk food, your body will spend most of its energy trying to process the junk and extract from it whatever little nutritional value it contains, thus creating more junk and weighing you down more and more. This results in speeding up the aging process.

We use food to make our own fuel. Fuel is energy. Before food can be turned to fuel, however, it must be broken down into very small particles that eventually become the raw ingredients of energy. This process is called *metabolism,* and it's under the direct control of our hormones. I'm sure you know (and probably hate) people with fast metabolisms who seem to immediately burn up every piece of cake they eat and never gain an ounce. I'm sure you also know and feel sorry for people with slow metabolisms, those unfortunate souls who get fat just by looking at a piece of bread. While genetics are important in determining who has a slow or fast metabolism, hormones are the real modulators. Patients with low thyroid are a well-known example of slow metabolism. Lesser known is that when estrogen and progesterone start waning, the metabolic rate slows down as well, and we start gaining weight. The connection between low thyroid and low estrogen and progesterone has only recently been made in conventional literature. Supplementation with estrogen and progesterone before treatment with thyroid medication is now being investigated. When we supplement with natural hormones, we prevent the metabolic slowdown. Of course, this isn't an excuse to eat junk food. We still need to make the right diet choices to maintain the body's ability to make clean and fast energy.

Your body turns food into energy in much the same way a refinery turns crude oil into high-octane gasoline. The wrong food will clog up the whole system and leave you feeling drained, exhausted, and very hungry. The right food will enhance your level of energy, leaving you satisfied, healthy, and full of vigor. Regardless of what you eat—a piece of chicken, a candy bar, or a great salad—the food will be broken down into the same tiny molecules to be used by the cells for energy production. These broken-down foodstuffs wind up as one of three basic substances—sugars (simple sugars), amino acids (building blocks of proteins), and fatty acids (building blocks of fats). It is these molecules that arrive at their final destination inside every cell of the body, into the mitochondria—the little factories inside the cells where energy is made and where all hormones start taking shape.

Metabolism encompasses the process of transforming food into energy and into building blocks for hormones. During this transformation, waste products known as toxins are created by the cells. This is normal and inevitable. The foods we eat either increase the amount of toxins we make or increase the amount of energy we produce. When our bodies are trying to make useful fuel out of foods that are highly processed, the cells become exhausted, and there's less energy available for hormone production and life enjoyment.

Balancing Your Foods

The first step in the process of fine-tuning your eating habits is understanding how to balance your food intake. We are taught in high school about the food pyramid. I would like you to think of the "food balance" instead. To achieve ideal nutritional intake, the balance should always be heavier on the side of protein and fiber, and lighter on the side of sugar and fat. Always aim to eat more protein and fiber— but don't forget your good sugars and fats, either.

Food Balance

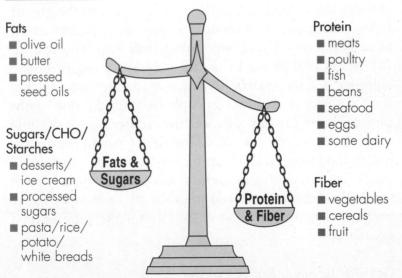

Fats
- olive oil
- butter
- pressed seed oils

Sugars/CHO/ Starches
- desserts/ ice cream
- processed sugars
- pasta/rice/ potato/ white breads

Protein
- meats
- poultry
- fish
- beans
- seafood
- eggs
- some dairy

Fiber
- vegetables
- cereals
- fruit

Fats & Sugars

Protein & Fiber

Natural Foods

When I talk about natural foods, I mean unprocessed, untreated foods. But this whole concept is at odds with the conveniences created by our modern age. How is it that we can have cereal in boxes that sit on grocery shelves for months, or canned foods that last for years? The answer, unfortunately, is preservatives. Laden with chemicals, our foods look good, taste wonderful, and create a faster-aging body. Our cells have no innate ability to deal with the processed, refined, and artificial foods that make up so much of our standard diet. While our taste buds have been corrupted by the preservatives in our foods, our cells can best digest and process only foods for which we have the right enzymes. And these foods are natural food substances without chemicals.

I tell my patients to just try eating unprocessed foods for a week or two. Invariably, they tell me about the remarkable changes they experience in their level of energy, the quality of their sleep, and their moods. So why aren't we all turning to natural foods? The answer I often hear is: "It's more difficult to get healthy food than a candy bar, a bag of potato chips, or a soda." Maybe that was true five years ago, but now, with more and more people becoming aware of the importance of eating good food, the excuse just doesn't hold water. Don't worry, I'm not asking you to run to the nearest health food store to stock up on organic, pure, nonsprayed foods. Even large chain supermarkets these days carry fresh foods, multigrain cereals and breads, nuts, fruit, and organic meats. Why not start there? You'll feel the difference! I guarantee it.

Get Off the Sugar Roller Coaster

Sugar might seem to give us the energy we're lacking in

the middle of the afternoon, or when we're about to get our period and progesterone and estrogen levels are dropping precipitously. But the price we pay for eating sugars is too high. Sugar—as in candy, candy bars, chocolate, cake, and indeed, sweets in general—turns into glucose the second it enters our bloodstream. Our blood sugar levels rise quickly. We feel a rush of energy; the shaky, sweaty, hungry feeling is gone. The problem is that the brain, seeing all this sugar bathing its cells, sends a message to the pancreas to release insulin. With the surge in insulin, the blood sugar level then drops, and every cell available uses up the sugar as though it were its last meal. Within a couple of hours, sometimes less, the insulin has left you drained of sugar, drained of energy, and back in the shaky, sweaty, hypoglycemic state you were trying to get out of when you first ate. You are on a never-ending roller coaster—the same foods that made you hypoglycemic to begin with are the quick-fix foods you crave.

The need to eliminate refined sugar from our diet cannot be overstated. Refined sugar—a modern dietary invention— stimulates the production of insulin by the pancreas. The higher the insulin level rises, the more aging damage occurs to the organs of the body, and the faster the blood sugar level drops. This translates into fatigue, weakness, shakiness, and foggy thinking. The sugar roller coaster leaves us drained and old before our time. Refined sugars in the form of cakes, cookies, ice cream, or pasta may taste delicious, but they're single-handedly our worst enemies in the fight against aging and the maintenance of hormone balance.

Fat Fads

Five years ago, low-fat diets were all the rage. After the connection between high cholesterol, heart disease, and diets high in saturated fats was made, physicians placed all patients at risk on low-fat diets. I was never keen on the idea, because I noticed that people who ate a very low-fat diet were always hungry, tired, and pasty, with thin hair and dry skin. Their cholesterol levels may have been low, but they sure looked and felt sick. The problem with low-fat diets in general is that they indiscriminately eliminate *all* fats from our diet. And fat is very important in the maintenance of our cellular membranes. It contributes to our having shiny hair, strong nails, and smooth skin, and it's essential for healthy brain and muscle function. Moreover, cholesterol is of utmost importance for the manufacture of estrogen— and it's the body's fat cells that store the estrogen we need when we get older and no longer manufacture it.

I'm not suggesting that we all start eating bacon, heavy cream, and fatty meats. The meat fats and most whole-dairy-derived fats are saturated—the culprits in our high-cholesterol, obesity, and heart disease problems. Another source of dangerous fats is margarine and hydrogenated oils. Called transfatty acids, they've been implicated in the increased incidence of heart disease and breast cancer our society is experiencing.

But the good fats—unsaturated fats—help maintain our youthful appearance and make hormone balance easier. (Women who have a few extra pounds do have an easier time with menopause.) You probably already know this. You know that after a meal full of saturated fats, you feel sluggish and start looking for a couch or a bed so you can take a nap. Not so with mono- and polyunsaturated fats. Not only do they keep your energy production up, but they also relieve PMS, decrease cholesterol, decrease blood pressure, decrease the risk of heart attacks, and may even decrease the growth of breast cancer.

Monounsaturated fats are found in olive oil, avocados, nuts, flaxseeds, and fatty fish. Health food stores and regular pharmacies all over the country sell these good fats in capsule form—look for linoleic acid (omega-6) and linolenic acid (omega-3). Adding them to your diet ensures that even if you're trying to lose weight, you can maintain the health benefits offered by a healthy-fat diet.

Weight Control

Any discussion dealing with nutrition and diet invariably ends in a conversation about weight loss. Obesity is at an all-time high in the United States. Everyone is looking for a quick way to lose weight. Half the women I see for hormone supplementation have come because they heard that natural hormone supplementation helps you lose weight. And while it does help, it's not a quick fix. You must watch your diet as well.

Most diets are based on the premise that if you put less food in your mouth (eat fewer calories), you'll force your body to break down its fat stores and lose weight. Not true. Indiscriminately going on a low-calorie diet will rob you of energy, will deplete your hormone levels, and—besides making you feel miserable—will not necessarily help you shed pounds. High-protein diets (the most extreme and destructive example being the Atkins diet) could strain your system and endanger the proper function of your kidneys and liver. And when you stop them, you will most likely rapidly gain all the weight back. Just as I successfully achieved symptom relief with natural hormones through a process of evolution, I developed the Hormone Solution Nutrition Program with the understanding that a successful diet can only be reached through balance.

Portions

Size matters.

To give your cells the ability to make good energy, maintain your hormones in balance, keep your blood sugar levels even, and keep insulin at bay, reasonable portions at frequent intervals are the most helpful tools. But don't go crazy measuring and weighing your foods.

One of my patients, a food critic, taught me to think about the way food is presented. She said that first you should imagine a beautiful plate in a great restaurant, then you must decide how much you should pile on it. If you want to lose weight, make it half of what you would ordinarily get served. If you want to maintain, make it three-quarters. But never make it a full plate, and be sure its presentation is appealing. Food that's not appealing to your senses will never be satisfying.

The Hormone Solution Nutrition Program

GROUP I:
PRELIMINARY SYMPTOMS
Age Group: Teens and early twenties

It would be unrealistic to expect teens to totally eliminate McDonald's french fries, tacos, or slices of pizza with soda from their diets. But unfortunately, some of the symptoms of hormone imbalance experienced by this age group are directly related to the highly refined sugar, saturated fat, and transfat content of the fast foods that are staples for people in their teens and early twenties.

Remember Michelle with the acne problem? Not only did she require topical antibiotics with natural progesterone supplementation to get rid of her acne, but she also needed a dietary makeover. She was a serious soda fan. She'd often have soda for breakfast, lunch, and dinner—and in between as well. When she felt a little tired, she'd take a swig of the soda she carried with her wherever she went. Over a period of two months, we weaned her off soda and taught her to drink water instead. While she still has her occasional soda fix, she drinks it only on special occasions now. This change in her diet was important. Soda is full of caffeine and sugar. These substances added insult to the injury of her hormone imbalance and most likely contributed to her problem with acne.

And recall Louise with the mood swings? It turned out she was a sugar addict, especially the week before her period. Her most severe mood swings coincided with nightly outings for frozen yogurt or ice cream. Not only did this pattern give her insulin problems, but the high sugar intake at night made it almost impossible for her to sleep. Natural progesterone cream helped tame her sugar cravings. Connecting the severe changes in personality to her nocturnal outings helped her stop the habit of the sugar fix. Louise still goes out for ice cream occasionally, only now she does it during the day and mostly on weekends.

Reasonable expectations is the rule for success in this group. They're young; they have to be given room to try different foods and enjoy life. But the sooner they learn to correlate symptoms to diet, the quicker they will feel better. Although teens should get help from their parents, it's important for them to learn to balance their diets on their own. You don't want them to have to play catch-up the way we had to.

Encourage a balanced diet high in proteins, vegetables, and fruit. As often as you can, sit down and have a complete family dinner with them. Set the example for them. Do not encourage them to go on crash diets or become obsessed with weight and body image. Teens learn by example. You know their friends will go out for fast food. That doesn't mean you should as well. Take them to the supermarket once in a while and buy good foods together. It may not happen immediately, but if you set the right example they will follow in your footsteps.

GROUP II:
ADULT SYMPTOMS
Age Group: Midtwenties to thirties

Remember Marcia with the postpartum depression? She stopped cooking for her family after she had her baby. As her depression worsened, so did her eating habits. Marcia ate one meal a day, if that much. Between caring for the baby and feeling exhausted, she spent her days dragging. No wonder: Her single meal usually consisted of cereal, fast food, or a frozen dinner. Needless to say, there was almost no nutritional value in what she ate. She ate infrequently, and the food was toxic to her system. Between the rapid drop in hormones (the aftermath of childbirth) and the lack of substantial nutrition, Marcia spent her life on the sugar roller coaster. Her insulin levels—either sky-high or low—were counterbalanced by blood sugar levels in constant flux.

With this type of diet, she was adding insult to the injury of her already stressed system.

Once she began the program in *The Hormone Solution*, Marcia started improving her eating habits. She liked eggs, so she returned to having egg sandwiches on whole-grain toast for breakfast. Lunch was a little trickier to introduce, but within a few weeks' time, she started to eat tuna or chicken salad. She felt better, her energy level increased, and with the help of natural hormones, her drive to feel better returned. Dinner once again became the main family gathering time, and Marcia started to cook—perhaps a nice piece of meat, or fish, along with a vegetable and a salad. Her husband—who'd grown used to grabbing a slice of pizza on his way home from work—happily switched to the home-cooked meals Marcia presented almost every night. As her diet improved, her mood improved. The final step was to get Marcia and her husband out on a date on Saturday night. It worked.

Not all twenty- and thirty-year-olds have this much difficulty with their diets. But many do. This is the time of life when hormones are usually well balanced, and proper diet will enhance our state of well-being. High protein (fish, fowl) and high fiber (lots of vegetables, salads, fruit, and nuts) should be the mainstay of the young person's diet. If work or other commitments interfere, I recommend balance. If you're eating too much fast food during the week, make a point of eating lots of vegetables and unprocessed meats on the weekend. There's no such thing as too much salad or too many vegetables. When in doubt, head for the green, leafy, dark-colored foods. They're rich in nutrients and add value to your life.

An aside about alcohol in your twenties and thirties. Partying is an important part of the social scene of young people. Yet while the young person's liver may be able to detoxify alcohol, the rest of the body can't. Sleep, brain function, and ability to concentrate are directly impaired by alcohol in the system. I am again suggesting that you practice moderation. Enjoy life, but keep in perspective how the balance of what you eat and drink affects you.

GROUPS III AND IV: PREMENOPAUSE AND PERIMENOPAUSE
Age Group: Thirty-five to fifty-five

Olga—the thirty-five-year-old with bloating, PMS, weight gain, and sore breasts—belongs in this group. Besides needing natural hormones, Olga needed some nutritional guidance as well. While a teen or twenty-year-old can get away with a less-than-perfect diet, the situation changes drastically as we age. At this point in our lives, our hormone production starts to diminish, and it therefore becomes imperative to take our diets more seriously. The best way to prepare for the time when hormones start to desert us is to follow a healthy diet from the time we're teenagers. But if this hasn't been the case for you, it's never too late to change your eating habits.

Olga ate irregular meals. She never had breakfast, drank lots of coffee, had lunch on the run between jobs and kids. She prided herself that dinner was a family affair: She and her children ate together at least three times a week. What they had for dinner was another story. Olga always prepared pasta, or potatoes, or rice with steak and an occasional salad. She proudly informed me that the steak was always grade A quality and low in fat. For dessert, Olga's daughter baked brownies or chocolate chip cookies. This feast might have been okay for a twenty-year-old once a week, but for Olga it was a prescription for disaster.

I cannot overstate the damaging effects of fluctuating sugar and insulin levels on the body. With Olga's hormones all over the map, her diet only worsened the problem. My advice to Olga was simple. Start eating small meals every three or four hours to balance your sugar level and prevent the insulin from spiking. Make those meals high in protein (egg whites, beans, fish, chicken, turkey, white unprocessed meats, nuts, soy) and in fiber (vegetables, nuts, fruit in small potions, oats, bran); limit the intake of saturated fats and sugars (including starches such as pasta, bread, rice, and potatoes). Make your evening meal small, so you can digest it fast and get to sleep easily. Avoid more than one cup of caffeinated coffee a day. (Beyond its stimulatory effects on the nervous system, caffeine increases breast tenderness and cyst production. It has also been linked to infertility and osteoporosis. So until its name is cleared, we don't need to gamble on its negative effects.)

Finally, Olga started drinking water. Coming from a generation that didn't know water served any purpose beyond cleaning up, Olga was shocked at the remarkable improvement in her skin tone and color once she started drinking four to six glasses of water a day.

Of course, natural hormone supplementation made Olga's change in diet easier to undertake, by decreasing her sugar cravings and improving her sense of well-being. And the change in diet in turn improved the effectiveness of the hormones and returned Olga to a younger, more vibrant woman.

For the large number of women who belong in this category, my advice is to evaluate your diet, make the changes necessary to feel better as early as possible, and don't deviate from your course all that often. If you do, gently glide back to the middle of the road and enjoy the improvement—it's always highly significant.

GROUP V:
MENOPAUSE AND POSTMENOPAUSE
Age: Fifty-five-plus

Donna, the fifty-seven-year-old with a family history of osteoporosis, and Sophie, the seventy-eight-year-old retired nurse, are examples of women in need of natural hormones who understood the importance of diet in their lives. They both ate balanced meals, high in protein and fiber and low in carbohydrates and fats. They stayed away from the processed meats and fast foods. They were in the group most likely to integrate proper nutrition into a healthy lifestyle. Still, they also need vitamins and supplements to further protect them from the damaging effects of aging.

My advice, although not limited to this group, is to supplement the diet with the following basic vitamins and supplements:

- Vitamin E—400 IU a day. An antioxidant, this vitamin protects against cancer, may decrease the risk of heart disease and stroke, and may improve memory.
- Vitamin C—1,000 mg a day. An antioxidant, this vitamin stimulates immune function, protects from recurrent urinary tract infections, and decreases the risk of atherosclerosis and stroke.

- Vitamin D—400 IU a day. Increases calcium absorption and strengthens bones.

- Folic acid—400 mcg–1 mg a day. Decreases fibrocystic breasts, relieves PMS, decreases the risk of colon cancer, and lowers homocysteine levels.

- Vitamin B_6—100 mg a day, and vitamin B_{12}—100 mcg a day. Relieve hot flashes, PMS, mood swings, and muscle cramps.

- Calcium—1,000 mg a day, preferably in divided doses after midday and in conjunction with vitamin D and magnesium. Builds bones, decreases the risk of colon cancer, stroke, and high blood pressure. May relieve PMS symptoms.

- Magnesium—400–600 mg a day with calcium. Relieves PMS and fatigue, helps build bones, decreases angina and palpitations, decreases incidence of depression.

- Zinc—25 mg a day with calcium. May protect against dementia and depression.

- Coenzyme Q 10—60–120 mg a day. This is the most potent antioxidant present in every cell in our body. It revitalizes the heart, stimulates energy production at the cellular level, and delays brain aging.

- L-carnitine—500–1,000 mg a day. A nonessential amino acid critical to the production of hormones and energy at the cellular level. It protects against blood clots, controls lipid levels, strengthens cell membranes, and makes red blood cells.

- L-glutamine—500 mg before meals. It stabilizes blood sugar levels and protects from insulin spikes. It works in conjunction with calcium to curb sugar cravings.

Before taking these supplements and vitamins, consult with your doctor. Although infrequent, interaction with medications does exist. I stress the importance of sharing this information with your physician, however, because achieving balanced health is a team effort.

EXERCISE

My mantra is: "Exercise should not be a source of stress in our lives."

Although we are constantly bombarded with information on the importance of exercise, we seem to miss the point that exercise is a highly personal enterprise. Not everyone can or will get off the couch and join a spinning class three times a week, and be happy or even do well. Whether you're twenty or seventy, no exercise program will work for you unless you understand your body and treat it with respect. Before you even consider getting involved in an exercise program, you need to evaluate your reasons for doing so.

Let's say you're overweight. Depending on your age, your body configuration, your genetic makeup, and your personality, a whole array of exercise options is available to you. Figuring out what fits your goal is half the battle. Staying on the program comes naturally if you see results within a reasonable period of time. "Reasonable" means two to four months of committed and consistent adherence to the program of your choice.

Unfortunately, when it comes to exercise there are no shortcuts. If you're serious about implementing significant change in your physical plant, the first step is to get educated. I promise you this approach will save you money and heartaches, not to mention potentially dangerous accidents.

To learn about appropriate options and discover what works best for you, consult a physician specializing in exercise physiology, a physical therapist, or an experienced trainer at a well-respected gym. Once you know how much activity you need to lose weight or just get into shape, you and the expert can together develop the right program for you.

Don't run out and buy the newest exercise fad video or attempt to follow routines described in magazines. They may not be right for you. You could get hurt or be so disappointed with the results that you give up on exercising altogether.

Melanie is a perfect example. When I first saw her, she was forty-three and had a small frame. Because her weight had never been an issue, athletics weren't on her radar screen in her youth. Melanie had a family history of osteoporosis, and being small boned and not very athletic, she was at high risk herself. That's why she came to see me. In addition to starting her on natural hormones, I strongly advised her to start an exercise program focused on increasing her muscle strength as soon as possible. Although we discussed the importance—not to be minimized—of a gentle transition from no exercise to serious strength building, Melanie decided to do it on her own. She bought a video promising almost immediate results in only twenty minutes a day. Anxious to get on with it, Melanie followed the advice in the video religiously for two weeks. And for good measure, she did it on a daily basis. When I saw her, as a result of an urgent call, she had pulled her lower back out and her left shoulder was so painful that she had to stop exercising. Melanie was not only in pain, she was discouraged.

Although she was ready to toss in the towel, I

wasn't. Gently focusing on stretching before starting the actual strength training, allowing recovery time between workouts, and varying types of exercises were the key ingredients of the program that finally worked for Melanie. You should see her arms now—she wears sleeveless shirts all summer long. Her bone density studies are excellent as well.

Genetics, Age, and Type of Exercise

Before you jump on the bandwagon of exercise, let's slow down a little and evaluate the key variables that will directly affect your chances for success.

If ignored, genetics will create a major stumbling block. I feel for women who tell me that no matter how hard they exercise, they remain overweight. When I ask about their family history, it seems that their mothers and sisters often have weight problems, too. The adage "genes rule" is most relevant when developing expectations for an exercise program. If you're 5 feet tall, weigh 130 pounds, and wear size 12, you will never be 5 foot 10, weigh 125 pounds, and wear size 2. While the shape of your body can be altered with plastic surgery—liposuction, implants, augmentations—your bone structure and tendencies toward weight gain in particular areas (hips, thighs, bottom) are genetically set in stone. So even if you do decide to get some help from the knife, genetics will fight you and return your body to its presurgery shape as soon as it can. This knowledge should not deter you from exercise or a little nip and tuck, though; it's meant only to help you develop more reasonable expectations. Make the best of what you have. Don't set yourself up for failure by trying to accomplish more than is humanly possible.

Which brings me to the next issue—your age. Although more and more people in their sixties and seventies are exercising on a regular basis, the type of exercise and results are different from those a younger person would see under the same circumstances. I marvel at the middle-age men I see who are fighting a constant uphill battle at the gym pumping iron next to cut twenty-year-olds. The older guys are pulling muscles, tearing ligaments, feeling worse with each routine, and blaming themselves for being inadequate while never addressing their age as the culprit. I realize they think that admitting that they're getting older could be translated into giving up, but I know that isn't necessarily the truth. It's about being realistic and thus protecting yourself from damage. Once you understand that aging changes your body's response to exercise, you can get involved in an exercise routine that will help you stay limber and strong practically forever. Be gentle to yourself and you'll find that even if you're eighty, you can still be in fine shape.

So, start slowly. Stretching becomes the most important part of any exercise program as we age. People who stretch on a regular basis, for a minimum of ten minutes before and after any significant physical activity, find themselves able to perform at the same level as people twenty years their junior. Warming up takes longer with age, but once the joints and muscles have been lubricated and put into gear, I'll match any sixty-year-old against a forty-year-old.

All too often, I meet women in their sixties who are reluctant to start exercising because they never did it before; they think they're too old. I believe you should start exercising as soon as you can walk, if not sooner, but by the same token I don't think you're ever too old to start. Just remember Melanie's experience, and pace yourself.

The type of exercise you choose is very important. Look at exercise as an investment in your future. If you start thinking long term, you'll quickly realize that the more variety of exercises you bring into your life, and the earlier in life you start, the more likely you are to prevent chronic illness and disability.

My mother died at eighty-six of natural causes. She was old, had beaten breast cancer five years before, and was tired. Remarkably, though, she exercised until the last month of her life. When she was in her sixties, she biked; in her seventies and early eighties, she took up swimming and water exercises; even in her mideighties, when she needed a walker to assist her, she still moved. This woman was never what you would call an athlete, but she always did something physical. Whether she planted flowers, walked up and down the street to say hello to her neighbors, or just did her daily sit-up and light weight routine, she never stopped moving. When she was in her late seventies, she moved into an assisted living complex. She quickly began a program for her neighbors that got many of them off the couches, away from the television sets, and out and about walking around the grounds every day. My mother may have been a bit ahead of her time in her commitment to preserving her ability to move and stay flexible and strong, but she certainly was successful and taught me right. Watching her over the years, I learned about the need to change types of exercise with advancing age. To this day, I remember her advice when prescribing exercise programs for my patients.

While it's great to join a team and become involved in track, field, or serious weight training in your teens and twenties, you must change in your thirties and forties to gentler, more focused, personalized exercise. Being in good shape doesn't mean you have to be a jock forever. Preparation starts in your teens, but persistent, consistent, and age-appropriate exercise will keep you active and vital through your later years.

The highlights of a successful approach to exercising for general groups according to age are summarized in the following paragraphs. Find your group and use the guidelines, but realize that the earlier you start and the more individualized your program, the more successful you'll be.

GROUP I
Age Group: Teens and early twenties

Our American educational system encourages physical activity. Every high school student takes physical education a few times a week, and many participate in some type of team sports. This is a great start. I advise parents to help their children stay focused and involved in team sports for as long as possible. Sociologic research has shown that children who stay involved in team sports through college are more disciplined, deal better with stress, and integrate into society more easily than their nonathletic counterparts. So what happens to those of us who don't go to college on an athletic scholarship? Most young adults rapidly fall into the trap of becoming overworked and finding little or no time for athletic endeavors. The time to develop a consistent and successful exercise program and make it a permanent part of your life is during your early twenties. I know it's a hard concept to sell, especially when you're young, weight is not an issue, age thirty seems far away, and no one even knows what *osteoporosis* means. Still, a physically active twenty-year-old has more energy, can concentrate better, and can fend off illness more than an inactive teen. And that is a fact.

Here are some general guidelines for the teens-to-twenties group that work and aren't difficult to integrate into everyday life:

- Engage in team sports.
- Try as many sports as you can. The more athletic endeavors you undertake as a youth, the better shape

your body will be in. Exposure to many sports will help you find the right ones as you get older.

■ Make exercise an integral part of your life. Don't let a day go by without including some type of physical activity. This is the time in life when you're building the foundation for later years. The same way you go to school to prepare for the future, if you can create a track record of always being physically active, you'll never get old.

GROUPS II AND III
Age Group: Late twenties to forties

This is the group of women who are having children, raising them, working full time. Exercise falls far behind as a priority now—yet the hormone changes we're undergoing during these critical decades will cause less stress if exercise is a constant in our life. Make time to exercise. As your body is changing due to childbirth, lifestyle, diet, and stress, your exercise program should adjust to these changes. Time taken to exercise at this point in life represents without a doubt a long-term investment in health in your later years. This is the time to formalize an all-inclusive program of aerobic exercise, weight and strength training, flexibility, and cardio fitness. If you do it right and do it now, you'll be healthy and fit for the rest of your life.

Here are basic suggestions for all to follow:

■ Join a gym and take an aerobic class three times a week.

■ Walk for half an hour every day carrying light weights (1 to 3 pounds).

■ Use exercise time to socialize. Play tennis; go swimming, hiking, mountain climbing, kayaking, or biking; participate in a team sport with your friends. Instead of going out to lunch or coffee, socialize while doing something physical.

■ Start and stay with a daily routine of strength building and stretching. At this point in life, you can build muscles easily: Starting with 3 to 5 pounds of weight, results can be obtained in six to eight weeks of consistent exercise. Repetitions of ten every other morning for ten minutes before getting into the shower should become part of your daily routine. Everyone has ten minutes to invest in health. Just think of it as any other routine, like brushing your teeth.

■ After thirty, stop high-impact aerobics, running, or jogging. *No jumping jacks.* They will increase wear and tear on your joints and precipitate prolapses of your uterus and bladder. You may not think it applies to you now, but the dribbles when you laugh and cough of the midfifties start right here in your thirties from too many jumping jacks and too much overenthusiastic high-impact aerobic exercise.

■ Do yoga once a week. Learn to incorporate relaxation and flexibility in your exercise routine. This is the time in life when learning how to deal with stress becomes very important. Properly employed relaxation techniques preserve your health and protect your body from injuries.

■ Have a monthly massage—try shiatsu or lymphatic drainage. A good massage improves your flexibility and removes muscle spasms, thus protecting you from injuries. When choosing a massage therapist, please be careful. Get information on his or her training and experience. Don't turn your body over to an inexperienced person, who can easily create more damage than help. If you have a massage and feel worse after it, don't go to the same person again. The rule of thumb should always be: "Feel better or reconsider."

■ Dance. Take ballet, line, ballroom, salsa, any dancing. It's a social sport good for your body *and* mind.

GROUPS IV AND V
Age Group: Late forties onward

If you've spent your whole life exercising on a regular basis, this time is simply another stage in your continuum of physical activity. Most of us are human, however, and spend our youth just taking our bodies for granted. Rest assured, it's never too late to start moving—and it's also never too late to reap the incredible benefits of an integrated exercise program. By that I mean diet, lifestyle, and exercise working together at all times to provide you with optimum vitality and health.

Natural hormones will help turn back the clock and give your body its best chance at staying young: Take advantage of this opportunity and avoid osteoporosis, heart disease, and debilitating chronic illnesses. Establish a daily routine that includes serious weight or resistance training, along with stretching and flexibility enhancement exercises.

In later years, our body isn't as forgiving as it was during our youth. It may be obvious, but somehow people don't seem to heed this important concept when addressing physical activity. When you're young, your body can take a serious amount of abuse and quickly recover. Older bodies can achieve high levels of stamina but require a significant warm-up period with stretching before getting into the main activity. The focus must be on maintaining flexibility and muscle strength.

Clark came to see me at the age of seventy-five. He looked twenty years younger and was an avid skier and tennis player. He wanted testosterone because his sex life had started to slow down, and he refused to give in to aging. Six months into the therapy with testosterone, Clark was doing very well. He even noticed improvement in his exercise endurance and muscle building. He felt rejuvenated and praised our program. Then one day he called to tell me he had pulled a muscle while skiing. A week later, he was on the slopes again—but this time he tore a ligament. I was baffled. Speaking with Clark at length, I solved the mystery. He thought he was forty again. Because he was doing so well on the testosterone, he started to skip warm-ups and cool-downs as part of his exercise routines. And he started getting injured.

The key to exercise in our older years is patience. If you take your time and warm up, stretch, and limber up before and after workouts, you can do as much as when you were younger. Once Clark realized that he would actually be protecting himself and accomplishing more by taking his time when exercising, he didn't get injured again. To this day, he's running down the slopes with the twenty-year-olds—the only difference is, he takes half an hour to warm up on his own before joining his younger pals.

Here are key differences to approaching exercise in our fifties through nineties to ensure success and avoid injuries:

- Before starting the day, stretch for twenty minutes. Get out of bed, get on the floor, and stretch. Do sit-ups, crunches, and weights (2 to 4 pounds). It doesn't matter how many, but it does matter that you stretch for the whole twenty minutes.

- Walk every day. The more you walk, the better you'll feel. Two miles is the least you should do.

- Take a Pilates class. Join other women your age and get involved in gentle exercising routines with the goal of stretching and building your flexibility and strength. Aerobic exercise in the sense of what you did at twenty or thirty is actually counterproductive and potentially harmful at sixty.

- Swim. Swimming is a great exercise. No pressure is applied to your joints when swimming, and your muscles become strong with practically no stress. People who live in warm climates can access swimming pools easily; in cold climates, swim at least during the summer months.

- Dance. Socializing and athletic endeavors work hand in hand. You won't age if you're physically and socially active. So what could be better than combining the two whenever possible?

- Get on a treadmill whenever possible and walk at 3.5 miles an hour and an incline of 2 percent for twenty minutes. It may not sound like much, but it will keep your arteries clear, and the consistency of the treadmill will give you all the cardio-aerobic exercise you really need.

- Bike, trek, canoe, ski, play tennis, go ice or in-line skating. Do everything you did at forty. Just do it after warming up, and remember to cool down afterward.

In the final analysis, the exercise program you undertake should be reasonable. Exercise should not be a drain or a chore; it should add to your sense of well-being and be something you look forward to. Exercise should not be just relegated to a method for losing weight: Your health depends on your moving. Moving means regular workouts, strength and flexibility training. Moving means never letting a whole day go by without undertaking some type of physical activity. I tell my patients all the time: "You don't need to change into workout clothes or go to the gym to get the physical activity your body needs. The opportunity to exercise exists every minute of your life. All you need to do is grab it."

- When you're driving your car, tighten your butt. Repeat ten times.

- When you're sitting at your desk at work, lift a paperweight and pump it ten times while on the phone. Or maybe just bring a 3-pound dumbbell to work and leave it on the floor by your desk. Grab a water bottle, use it as a weight, then drink it. You can get a lot done without stressing or preparing.

- When you get up in the morning, get on the floor and do twenty sit-ups before you take your shower.

- Park your car at the farthest point in the parking lot and walk to your destination.

- Don't take the elevator—walk up those steps. Even if you're heading to the fifth floor.

You don't have to be a jock to reap the benefits of physical activity for the rest of your life. Whether you're twenty or seventy, strength and flexibility translate into youth and health. Vigor and energy are directly related to the amount of movement you include in your life. And as you get older, strength and flexibility become more important. If you have strong muscles, you won't get osteoporosis, regardless of your genetic makeup.

LIFESTYLE

We all live in a stressful world. To deny it is to add more stress.

Learning to identify our stressors and then dealing with them is a more reasonable option. Natural hormones are a wonderful, gentle way of balancing your hormones, but they cannot work in a vacuum. No treatment can work if your lifestyle is counterproductive and destructive to your body and mind.

Linda was a forty-seven-year-old nurse. She was very knowledgeable about hormones, so when she started experiencing too many symptoms of hormone deficiency, she came to see me to start a combination micronized progesterone and estradiol in a cycled program. I saw her once a month for two months. She did not feel better. Her hot flashes diminished and her night sweats were almost gone, but overall Linda was not well. I went over her diet and exercise regimens with a fine-toothed comb. She was nothing short of perfect. At my wit's end, I asked her to talk to me about her personal life. As it turned out, Linda was in trouble.

A ten-year relationship with a man had ended abruptly a few weeks before her hormone troubles started. She was afraid to tell her friends, her coworkers, her family. So she hid. She made excuses and stayed home. The stress in Linda's life was mounting. She saw no way out. No wonder the hormones weren't helping her! Nothing could. Linda went into therapy. A couple of months later, she started telling everyone the truth—and her symptoms disappeared.

Very often, complaints that bring symptoms of hormone imbalance to the surface are precipitated by major life changes. To ensure the success of a treatment plan, you cannot ignore your lifestyle.

De-stress

Unrelenting stress is the greatest energy zapper known, and a large impediment to the successful treatment of medical and mental conditions.

The only solution is to de-stress. Of course, that's easier said than done. Everything we do stresses our system. Whether it's mental stress from life's tragedies, family issues, personal losses, or work-related challenges, or physical stress in terms of eating, rest, and exercise patterns, the result is wear and tear on the whole system.

This wear and tear cannot be eliminated, but it can be delayed and minimized.

Hormone balance plays an enormous role in our ability to tolerate stress. But even when that balance has been achieved, we must identify the stressors to which we're particularly vulnerable as individuals and figure out if we can do something about them. When you feel under significant pressure, get a diary and write the events that precipitated your feelings.

My young women patients find out very quickly that before they get their periods, they feel stressed. School, work, family ties become unbearable; they feel ready to snap. While progesterone cream certainly abates the snapping feeling, the reality of being a teen still exists and must be dealt with. The same thing goes for the forty-seven-year-olds who cannot juggle work, family, and friends any longer. Hormones help, but dealing with the problems and making them less stressful is an absolute must. Stress solutions:

■ Put it in an imaginary drawer and shut it! Face your biggest problem. If you can't do anything about it, just put it into an imaginary drawer and shut it. We're accustomed to working out every problem, struggling with it until we find a solution. Some problems don't have solutions, at least for a while; rather than stressing yourself when there's no answer to be found, give yourself a break.

■ Take a deep breath out! A good friend of mine once gave me a great tape by an Eastern master. I listened to it a few times. I knew I would never become a yoga devotee, but I learned an important piece of advice from the tape: When I feel overwhelmed, I stop and take a deep breath *out!* Somehow when you breathe in, you are bringing into your body all the stress and worry from the outside world. When you breathe out, though, all the stuff you held in just dissipates into the outside. It may not make my problems go away, but my load becomes more tolerable.

■ Pause, even for a second! In tennis, the difference between an average and a good tennis player is timing. A split-second delay allows you to focus better and see where the ball is going, how to better hit it, and how to direct your shot. Take this split-second delay concept and apply it to your life. Before reacting in a stressful situation, take a deep breath out—then stop for a split second. In this moment you can consider whether your reaction is worth having, or if there are better ways to deal with the situation. The split-second delay allows you to become aware of yourself and your surroundings. The message is: Don't react blindly. I'm not recommending you start intellectualizing everything and lose the spontaneity that makes you unique. Just stop for a split second and think about what you really should do.

■ Stop feeling stuck in the past! Linda's story is a perfect example of this type of stressor. When something happens that you have no control over, let go of it. Be sad, mourn the situation, but holding on to it and trying to make believe it didn't happen or that you could have changed its outcome will only make your stress level go up. I find many male patients who invariably stay stuck in their youth. They believe their best days are behind them—high school football, college swimming, their twenties. If you believe the best is in your past, then that will be true. Instead, look at today and how you can make the future better. Get the most out of today instead of spending your precious energy on yesterday.

■ Take one step at a time! Much of the time, my life is overwhelming because I find myself biting off more than I can chew. I don't know how to say no. Unfortunately, I found out the hard way that if I do less, I accomplish more and leave a lot less disappointment behind. Start saying no once in a while. You'll stay focused and move ahead faster. Give up on doing twenty things at once.

■ Communicate! Clearing up misunderstandings is probably one of the least addressed lifestyle issues. We are all so afraid of confrontation, of being perceived as a bully, that we allow miscommunication to ruin our lives. Do you find yourself in the same discussions and arguments over and over again with certain people in your life? Do you leave meetings and conversations feeling you weren't heard or understood? How often do you wonder what the person you were talking to was trying to say? Poor communication skills are at the root of this problem. Often when people talk, they're so busy preparing their answer and wanting to get their point across that they don't listen to the other person. The result is a stressed and frustrated human on both sides of the conversation. So don't waste precious energy; take the time to listen and relax enough to allow another point of view to filter through. As a result, you will be carrying less on your shoulders—and the world will be an easier place to be in.

■ Have reasonable expectations! When patients come to see me for the first time, I always wonder what their expectation level is. It's a very important barometer of the type of person I'm dealing with and a strong indicator of how he or she will respond to the therapy. The one extreme is the woman who wants to walk out of the office with hormone creams in hand (even though they have to be individually prepared in a pharmacy at some distance from the office) and start treatment today. The other extreme is the woman who—after spending time and money on an extensive consultation with me, laboratory testing, formulation of the hormones, and reading of the educational materials— spends the next two months thinking about when to stop her Premarin and start the new regimen. Fortunately for all, most people fit somewhere in the middle. I always fear that the extremists will be disappointed, because their expectations aren't reasonable. Be realistic. I tell my new hormone patients, "Let's give it three months. Let's balance, change the dosing, and talk about it once a month or more often if necessary. But begin with the premise that it will take three months to reach a good balance." In fact, most people take less time than this, but I cut myself and the patients some slack. I don't feel overly pressured, and the patients are invariably pleasantly surprised. The same is true for the rest of your life.

- Get a new attitude! The most important de-stressor may be simply changing your own outlook. Take the attitude that life is as good as it gets. Rather than always looking to improve the future or blaming yourself for the past, learn to treat yourself kindly now, in this moment. I'm not referring to the obligatory manicure, the massage and facial, or the trip to the mall; I mean something simpler. Give yourself permission to be you, to be who you really are. Give yourself permission to age, but not to give in. If you're fifty, don't try to be thirty; just be the best fifty you can be for yourself. Don't use anyone else's standards: Define yourself as the unique person you are. Take responsibility for your life and either accept it as it is or change it for the better with your new attitude.

- Engage! I get very nervous when I see aging women who are depressed. Hormones will make them feel better, but to what end? The kids grown, the husband may not be present either, women who are isolated are at risk. Boredom is a dangerous mind-set. Get out of the house; join a club, a church, a charity; get a job. Boredom is a place we go to hide from our feelings and our problems. Your mind knows that if you address the reality of your situation, you have to do something about it—so it shuts down. Don't let it! Use a diary to see what's really going on in your life. The entries will show you where you are and if you're hiding from troublesome reality spots.

■ Retirement is a danger spot for most active people. Andrew, a construction worker patient of mine, became more and more of a couch potato over a period of six months after his retirement. His wife brought him to me for testosterone supplementation because she thought he was depressed. Testosterone improved his libido, but it didn't get him off the couch. I suggested he start walking every day. He said his arthritis was bothering him too much. I suggested he go to church with his wife on Sunday. He couldn't; the service conflicted with his favorite Sunday-morning news show. I told him to tape the show and just go to church. He reluctantly agreed. The minister must have heard my prayers, because he asked Andrew to help supervise a construction project at the church. Andrew got off the couch and went back to work. Now he even walks to church and bought a treadmill for his basement. See what a little engaging can do?

■ Sleep! I addressed the relationship between sleep disorders and hormone imbalance in chapter 3, but I want to reinforce its significance. Sleep is sacred. If you don't get it, you get cranky, your focus is off, you get sick, and your hormones become confused and out of sync.

Sleep is so critical for hormone production that it cannot be overstated. When the hormones are in balance and we can sleep, we must ensure that other factors do not deter us from sleeping, because sleep is equivalent to youth. If you sleep well, you live longer.

Here are some tips to help improve your chances for a good night's sleep—with the assumption that your hormones are in good balance:

- Clear your bedroom of things that don't belong there: All work papers must go. Draw the shades; keep the room cozy and uncluttered.

- Eliminate the TV. Either remove it from your bedroom or just make sure it's off when you go to sleep. Do not leave the TV on. The sounds and light from it will continue to enter your brain, and the quality of your sleep will be diminished. Television is the single most common deterrent to sound sleep.

- Watch the timing of your last meal. Eating a heavy dinner late will interfere with good sleep. Go to sleep lighter, and you'll sleep sounder. Alcohol does not improve sleep quality. It may help you fall asleep faster, but it will also wake you up earlier, and your sleep will be restless and unsatisfying.

- Don't exercise too close to bedtime. Those wonderful endorphins that make us feel good when we exercise are also going to stop us from getting the deep sleep we need to renew ourselves. So don't exercise within two hours of going to sleep.

And for my final advice: A little at a time will change your whole life in no time. Be nice to yourself. You are unique; celebrate your uniqueness, don't hide it. If you're tired, sleep. Things will wait. If you're sad, cry. You'll feel better. When you're happy, enjoy. Others will enjoy with you.

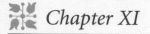 *Chapter XI*

What About Men?

$\mathcal{M}$artha, a patient and a friend who is forty-eight, got married last year. She found the right guy. He adores her, she worships him, they have fun together, and they cope well with all the kids and exes in their lives. Martha tells me that Mark is very loving, and she's never been happier. But while she's on the Hormone Solution Program and is going through her changes with no problems, Mark seems to be having some trouble. At times, Mark's mind says yes but some of his body isn't listening—his erections seem to be flagging. They tried Viagra, which helped, but they're worried about the potential dangers of the drug. Martha doesn't want Mark to have a heart attack, and she doesn't like unnecessary medication in his body. It took too long to find him.

His erection problem isn't the only concern. His once-buff body isn't so buff anymore. He goes to the gym, still pumps iron—he always looked great—but at fifty something has changed: He's getting a little soft in the middle, even a bit of a beer belly. He thought there was no solution—just aging. Everyone gets this way in their forties and fifties. Then he read an article about the increasing use of testosterone supplementation in middle-age men in the *New York Times Magazine,* and immediately took it to his doctor. Unfortunately for Mark, his doctor said he doesn't believe in information disseminated through consumer channels. He gets his information only from medical journals and pharmaceutical people, and he's not comfortable with testosterone supplementation. Middle-age males' erections are not his specialty, thus he seldom reads journals with a focus on "male plumbing." So much for help from this doctor! (I wonder how old Mark's doctor is? Maybe he'll get more interested when he starts having problems with his own erections.)

Martha brought Mark to see me, and I started him on micronized testosterone cream. After a couple of months, remarkable changes came over him. He lost some of his beer belly and started to feel rejuvenated when he saw his musculature return to its prior shape. And Martha tells me he's now chasing her around the house, the way he did when they first got together.

The role of male hormones is at the same time extremely important and baffling. Our culture bombards us with reminders of how different men and women are. Not only do we think differently, many would have us functioning differently on a physiologic level as well. Yet we have the same internal organs—the same mechanisms to make our hearts beat, to breathe air in the lungs, to digest the food we eat, and to excrete the waste we create. Why would men and women be different when it comes to the hormone depletion that we've unequivocally established is associated with aging?

When I became involved with the study of hormones, I never thought in terms of men. My involvement was mostly based on personal experience and need. I wanted a safe solution for my personal symptoms of hormone deficiency, and by association I found solutions for my female patients. I did not address men, but that was an error. No sooner did I focus my clinical practice on natural hormone supplementation for women than the women started to talk about and bring in their men.

※

When I first started practicing medicine, my knowledge about male hormones came largely from the education I received in medical school. That was in the 1970s, and although I went to a progressive medical school, it was still a time when hormones were not a well-researched or popular topic. We were taught very little more than "testosterone is the main male hormone."

And without any doubt, testosterone is the hormone that differentiates men from women. It's made in the testicles and is responsible for the production and multiplication of healthy sperm. Secondary sexual characteristics occur as a direct result of testosterone flooding a boy's system in early puberty. Testosterone makes his voice change, makes body and pubic hair grow, gives perspiration its typical pungent male odor, makes the penis and the testicles grow to adult size, makes men physically stronger than women, and enables them to develop beautifully sculptured bodies shortly after starting a regular workout program. And yes, testosterone is probably responsible for the way men think and process problems. And there my basic education on testosterone ended.

What followed in my medical school course about male endocrinology was a series of syndromes and illnesses associated mostly with testosterone deficiency. Oddly enough, they all seem to occur in young men, unlike the later timing of the appearance of hormone problems in women. Once you made it through puberty and adolescence, brought down undescended testicles, treated the rare case of testicular cancer, dealt with an occasional inflammation or infection of the foreskin, or addressed poor sperm motility in infertile men, *testosterone* very much disappeared from the medical vocabulary. And even more oddly, it never returned.

TESTOSTERONE TODAY

I rarely heard the terms *male menopause* or *andropause* until around five years ago. In my extensive research on hormones, I never read an article decisively connecting male hormone deficiencies with symptoms of midlife. Looking back over the past sixteen years I've spent in private practice, I wonder why my profession has overlooked the possible relationship between men's midlife problems and hormone deficiency syndromes. We are certainly ready to admit that men do experience midlife problems; so why are we missing their connection to testosterone levels? What is midlife crisis really all about?

Male menopause is technically known as andropause, or male climacteric. The reason andropause has never been in the public spotlight is that men who experience it have been reluctant and unwilling to acknowledge its existence. Somehow the decrease in testosterone levels that naturally occurs in men during middle age has remained a little-known fact. I don't know why it should be so surprising to acknowledge that men are physiologically similar to women. Just like women, when men start aging, their hormones start to decline as well. Symptoms of hormone insufficiency in men present quite often, and closely resemble symptoms of hormone insufficiency in women. The middle-age gut, the couch potato stance, the depression associated with men in their middle years are all clear and unequivocal symptoms of the decline in testosterone levels. Look at the man in his fifties who is unsuccessfully trying to build muscle mass. Yes, he's aging, but it's his decreasing testosterone levels that make him ineffective when he tries to build muscle mass. It's not that he suddenly just stopped trying.

Unfortunately, the medical profession has not been keen on addressing this obvious similarity to female menopause. Most doctors are men, and *menopause* does not have a pretty ring to it—it's about aging. And men are more afraid than women to address the inevitability of this process. Men pride themselves on the ability to father children into their eighties, so how could they be having the same problems as aging women? (The truth, by the way, is that men who father children naturally in their eighties are as rare as women who give birth in their fifties.)

As women started to openly address their issues with hormone deficiencies in the 1990s, an interesting paradox occurred. Although not immediately acknowledged as a problem, the issue of the decline in sexual performance encountered by many middle-age men moved to a more visible position as well. Maybe it's not as prominently displayed in the mass media, but nonetheless its presence has begun to be felt in the medical community. Of course, researchers have been studying male andropause for decades, along with the effects of reduced levels of testosterone in the aging process. It was the pharmaceutical companies however, that first saw a need among the population of aging men. Unfortunately, the direction the early solution took was synthetic, and it addressed one isolated symptom and not the root cause of the male andropause problem. By approaching the problem from the angle of one symptom only, the larger issue of male menopause could be easily sidestepped; it retained its place in the closet of male problems.

Before the issue of male menopause would even be acknowledged, the treatment for impotence was flooding the market.

VIAGRA

Viagra came onto the market like gangbusters. It carried a resounding message: "Our manhood is at risk, we have a problem with erections, and we are going to correct it quickly before anyone gets a chance to take a closer, more in-depth look at what is really going on with our aging men."

So Viagra moved into our consciousness. Practically every middle-age patient in my practice called asking for prescriptions for Viagra. I learned about it from the media and a Pfizer pharmaceutical representative who came to my office with free samples of the new magical drug. It was odd: One day impotence was never mentioned; the next it was the hottest topic of conversation from Wall Street to the kids on Main Street.

Although I'm very open minded, I was hesitant to write the prescriptions. I had nothing against the quick fix Viagra promised men, but I was worried that the wrong man would take it and become mortally ill from it. My fear came from the understanding of how Viagra works. It increases the blood flow to the penis and the pelvic organs in general. It brings more blood to the penis and, as a result, a harder erection. Great, exactly what we all want, but at what cost? If the man is older and has high blood pressure or heart failure, Viagra, by diverting blood from the heart, lungs, and brain, will induce a rapid drop in blood pressure to the organs that need the blood flow the most. This increases the risk for strokes and heart attacks. I didn't want to scare anyone, but I discouraged older men who had atherosclerotic disease from using it. Unfortunately, the very reason for their erectile problems was that they had plaque (athero-sclerosis) in the blood vessels supplying the penis to begin with. They were the men on medications for high blood pressure and cholesterol. They were also suffering from impotence, the most disturbing side effect of antihyperten-sive medication. A Catch-22 situation: The men who need the medication the most are at highest risk of getting complications from it.

Still, despite the dilemma of its side effects, Viagra had opened a new door. Its sheer existence acknowledges fairly prominently that men experience significant and disturbing problems as they age.

Men need help, too.

MALE HORMONES AND SEX

To feel sexual interest, you need hormones. When men pass from their midthirties into their midforties, they undergo significant changes. Their hormone levels, starting with testosterone, start to dwindle. Since men never talk about hot flashes and night sweats, we never knew they experience them. But they do. Many women patients are starting to talk about their men's night sweats, their mood swings, their depression, and their weight gain. And why not? Just as in women, male hormones do drop with age. Testosterone made in the testicles and adrenal glands starts waning with age, and as with women, when its quality and quantity decline, symptoms arise.

A few years ago the medical literature, and in particular journals of urology, started to publish articles connecting an improved sense of well-being in aging men on testosterone supplementation. It was a major step forward for a profession in which testosterone was used only to treat young males with diseases of hormone deficiency. It was a first step toward acknowledging the existence of male menopause. The connection between low testosterone levels and previously unaddressed and disconnected symptoms was being made by both the lay public and conventional medicine.

Finally, in the past three years, testosterone supplementation has entered the conventional world of wellness and anti-aging. It has not yet moved into the mainstream of medicine, however, or become a topic of dinner conversation the way menopause has. Men have started to admit to experiencing the same symptoms previously reserved to women, but the door is only slightly ajar. In my practice, in response to this growing need, I developed the Hormone Solution Program for Men.

George is a forty-seven-year-old retired policeman. He loves to read, tend his garden, and play with his grandchildren. George became depressed five years ago when an injury he experienced at work forced him to retire. He saw a psychiatrist and was placed on an antidepressant. The medication never worked, but George stuck with it. His mental condition deteriorated, and any medication the psychiatrist added only made matters worse. George developed severe mood swings; his sex drive disappeared. One night he saw a TV segment on testosterone on the local news. The doctor interviewed recommended the hormone for the treatment of depression in middle-age men. I saw George shortly thereafter. His wife brought him to me because his own doctor did not want to give him a prescription for testosterone. As part of the Hormone Solution Program for Men, I started him on a combination of testosterone cream and a diet and exercise program specifically aimed at improving his mood and stamina. Four months later, George discontinued the use of the antidepressants and had no recurrence of depression or mood swings.

Sidney is a large man. He weighs 235 pounds, stands 6 foot 5 inches tall, and was sixty-five years old when I first saw him. His wife, Lara, a petite 5-foot, 100-pound, forty-three-year-old, appears tiny next to her man. They came to see me together. She was going through hormone changes and he came along for moral support. They were recently married. Their sex life before the wedding was wonderful; they felt like teenagers. But soon after, something changed. Lara lost interest in sex, and Sidney's sex drive took a nosedive as well. And that was not all, he had been a bodybuilder, but now he was having trouble keeping his muscle mass. Needless to say, these problems caused him significant angst. I tested them both for blood hormone levels. While Lara's hormones were within normal limits, Sidney's testosterone was practically nonexistent. His PSA—reflecting the function of his prostate gland—was normal. I included Sidney in the Hormone Solution Program and also started him on micronized testosterone, 20 mg/day. Two months later, their sex life returned to normal and he no longer complained about muscle-building problems.

Every day one of my women patients brings up the topic of male menopause, or andropause. The question invariably is, "How can I help my husband/lover?" The answer is clear and simple and backed by numerous medical publications:

"Supplement his testosterone." So why aren't more doctors prescribing it? Do doctors still consider testosterone outside the area of conventional medicine? For our sake and our men's sake, I hope not. What used to be the domain of body-builders and athletes is now without a doubt a normal part of any man's world. To provide the proper solutions to men, conventional medicine must follow.

Before we go on, let's pause and look at the most common symptoms associated with testosterone depletion in the average, healthy, fifty-year-old man:

- Inability to build muscle as easily as at age twenty.
- Problems losing weight as easily as at age twenty.
- Inability to ejaculate as often as at age twenty.
- Problems maintaining an erection as long as at age twenty.
- Diminished sex drive.
- Depression and loss of excitement about life and career.
- Insomnia and other sleep disorders.
- Having to urinate at least once a night.
- Lack of energy.

Even if these symptoms don't appear to be exactly the same as those experienced by women as a result of hormone depletion, they're strongly similar. Beyond this point, though, women and men are not dissimilar in the expression of these deficiencies.

Just like women, certain men suffer from symptoms, incapacitating to various degrees, while some sail through this period of their life with minimal problems and settle into the next stage without much trouble. Those who do have difficulties are easy to identify. Just like their female counterparts, these men's lives are turned upside down. Coping mechanisms fail; the aging process becomes unmanageable.

Allen came to see me in a state of quiet desperation. He was a successful fifty-two-year-old attorney. His life had been on an even keel. When he turned fifty, though, things started to unravel. He stopped enjoying work, he had difficulties with family and friends, and he even stopped playing golf, his favorite hobby. His wife suggested he see a psychiatrist. The psychiatrist spent a long time talking to Allen, finally deciding to start him on Prozac. Allen felt a little better. He seemed to regain some of his lost joie de vivre, and even returned to his Saturday-morning golf game.

But something still wasn't right. The psychiatrist raised the dose of Prozac, and added another antidepressant for better balance (Wellbutrin). Allen became groggy; what little sex drive he had disappeared. His wife, also a patient of mine on the Hormone Solution Program, was coping well, and Allen's problems were a source of worry to her. One day, at work, Allen lost his temper and spun out of control. During an important meeting, he started screaming and acting totally out of character. Embarrassed, he apologized to his boss, and that same evening asked his wife to get him help. She brought him to me. I tested Allen's PSA, thyroid function, and testosterone levels. His testosterone level was very low. He was depressed and anxious at the same time. The medications prescribed to him were clearly not helping him, but only confusing an already difficult situation. After an extensive consultation, I started Allen on the Hormone Solution Program, including transdermal testosterone cream; we checked his blood hormone levels every six weeks. By the time his testosterone levels started to climb, Allen felt good enough to stop taking antidepressant medications. It only took two months to get Allen back to the life he thought he'd lost.

Allen's story is common for men in their forties and fifties who start taking testosterone supplementation. The unfortunate exceptions are the men who don't know about the miraculous recoveries achieved through testosterone supplementation. Because they don't know about the testosterone solution, they either ignore bothersome and destructive symptoms, or take antidepressant medications prescribed by physicians unfamiliar with the benefits and safety of the testosterone option.

TESTOSTERONE TESTING

When I started seeing men in need of testosterone supplementation, I couldn't find any clinical guidelines for dosing or systems of administration in the medical literature. Interestingly, in the general field of wellness, testosterone was first recognized as the feel-good hormone *women* could use to maintain and improve their sex drive in their forties and beyond. Although testosterone is *the* male hormone, little is reported on its use in men for similar purposes, in either conventional or alternative medical literature. Rare articles in the scientific journals reflect a sense of surprise when men treated with their own hormone for impotence, depression, and involutional melancholia react well to testosterone. In

July 2000, Dr. Jay Adlersberg of WABC-TV reported that more than four million men in the United States suffer from low testosterone. He added that low testosterone can cause "impotence, depression, and fatigue." His report concluded with patient testimonials praising the remarkable results of testosterone supplementation. After six months in the study, the participants reported increases in lean body mass, sex drive, and energy levels.

Similar to the situation with women, men's testosterone levels are not routinely measured when they undergo routine physical examinations. In those unusual cases where the levels are measured, the value considered normal is variable and the range quite broad, so most levels are deemed within normal limits.

This returns diagnosis of problems back to the area of clinical judgment of subjective symptoms: how the man feels.

But the road to finding solutions is a lot steeper for men. *Andropause* and *male menopause* are still dirty words in our society. As with women, different men experience different symptoms. Most don't have incapacitating hot flashes and night sweats. They don't have periods, which means we can't choose a point in time to pin "The Change" on. Diagnosing hormone deficiencies in men thus requires more detective work. And just think of how long it took women to start talking about menopause openly! No wonder men are so far behind in this area. Still, there's no reason to give up or continue ignoring the existence of andropause. Men need help with hormones just as much as women do.

And the payoff is just as high.

ADMINISTRATION OF TESTOSTERONE SUPPLEMENTATION

One of significant drawbacks to testosterone supplementation has been its method of administration. Testosterone can't be given by mouth, because it doesn't get absorbed from the stomach. For years, the only way to administer it was by injection—which is unreasonably invasive and painful. Most men would rather have symptoms of hormone depletion than take a shot every day or once a week. No wonder testosterone supplementation didn't become popular with the public at large! For years, it was reserved for the very young and the very ill.

Finally, a patch called Androderm was developed. Initially, it was used by men with testosterone deficiency diseases or AIDS-related malnutrition. Bodybuilders quickly followed—and women, too. Androderm did not make a big splash with middle-age men. Medical drawbacks abounded: too many skin reactions, unpredictability of absorption, and often increased aggressive behavior. The dosing is rigid, and absorption is unpredictable because the patch stays on your skin for days. It holds a small reservoir of testosterone and the amount released is variable. Another problem with the use of Androderm by healthy people is aesthetics. Wearing a patch is unsightly; many men and women find that it detracts from feeling sexy and remove it during sex. This makes its reliability even poorer, and its cost becomes prohibitive.

In 2000, Androgel (1 percent testosterone gel) came to the market. The FDA approved it for "treatment of low testosterone levels linked to decreased sex drive, impotence, reduced lean body mass, decreased bone density, and lowered mood and energy levels." The once-daily topical gel was not evaluated in women or men with prostate or breast cancer.

Androgel is a synthetic form of testosterone (methyltestos-terone) in gel form, with good absorption but rigid dosing. Androgel is superior to Androderm because its method of administration is more appealing, and the absorption better.

In an article published in January 2001, *Internal Medicine World Report* reported on the successful use of testosterone in pellet form. This method involved insertion of testosterone under the skin, in three to six 200 mg pellets that provided adequate testosterone supplementation for four to six months. The article reflected the results of an exhaustive nineteen-year Australian study involving men between the ages of twenty-four and sixty-seven. Beneficial results of testosterone involved more than its effects on enhanced sexuality and muscle mass—the study also raised the possibility of positive cardiac effects on the men who participated.

Another form of administration is micronized testos-terone. Like natural estrogen and progesterone, this form of supplementation is sold directly to pharmacists in powder form and is mixed to the doctor's specifications. This is superior to standard pharmaceutical methods because the dosage can be individually altered by the prescribing physi-cian. It's of great value to the patient because it addresses the individual's needs and not statistically determined dosages. Androderm, Androgel, and pellets are rigidly dosed; the doctor has little input as to the adjustment of each patient's dosage. They're also synthetic preparations of the hormone. Micronized testosterone is a natural base formulation. (It is the only kind of testosterone I use for my patients.) The patients who follow the Hormone Solution Program experi-ence a rapid, gentle rise in their testosterone levels with remarkable effects and exquisite safety records. The method of application, which is in cream form, is gentle and com-fortable. A specifically designed amount is rubbed into the skin of the inner thigh or on the scrotum once or twice a day. The dosage is easily adjusted using this method: The gauge is a combination of symptom relief and close monitoring of testosterone blood levels.

Testosterone is available by prescription only. Some states further supervise its use by classifying it as a controlled substance. That's because it is being recklessly used by bodybuilders. Androgel and Androderm patches can be obtained at any regular pharmacy, or the hormone can be individually compounded in its micronized form by compounding pharmacies.

The Hormone Solution Program successfully integrates individualized dosing of micronized testosterone with diet, exercise, and lifestyle in a comprehensive, medically supervised fashion to treat the whole man's needs. I strongly advise you to talk to your doctor and together evaluate your particular situation. Once the diagnosis of testosterone deficiency is made, you owe it to yourself to get the best preparation for you. Work with your doctor and find the type of supplementation best suited for your symptoms and lifestyle.

Final Words

The Hormone Solution represents a compilation of a lifetime of wisdom and twenty-seven years of my personal clinical experience and medical expertise. It is my mission statement. It arose initially from a need to find concrete, safe, and definitive solutions to my own hormone problems. As a woman and a practicing physician, I quickly realized that I couldn't find a satisfactory solution for the overwhelming and destructive symptoms produced by hormone imbalance by using the tools my conventional medical training offered. When I turned to alternative options, the results were no better. The treatments available in the area of hormone imbalance are an open wound for both conventional and alternative practitioners. No mass-produced solution has proven effective to date.

All scientists agree: Hormones are the common thread that makes up the fabric of our lives. They define us as men and women when we're young, they keep us healthy or make us sick, and yet the understanding we have of them is vague, contradictory, and inconsistent. Many researchers and clinicians allude to the connection between hormones and PMS, postpartum depression, mood swings, sexual dysfunction, migraines, weight gain, infertility, and even sleep disorders. Yet few take this important knowledge to the next level. Authoritative affirmation that hormones are the root cause of these symptoms, regardless of age, is lacking. Unequivocally, the scientific community knows that hormone levels change every minute of the day, so why get hung up on one or two changes: menopause and puberty? A small step for science, a giant step for women. Once you make that connection, once you identify the continuum of hormone changes, menopause is a lot less scary, and its devastation just another small mountain to scale.

If I hadn't become sick with hot flashes and night sweats and experienced the devastating side effects of conventional medications myself, I wouldn't have looked for a solution or written this book. If I hadn't spent thousands of dollars on herbal remedies without experiencing relief, I wouldn't have been motivated to search for a better solution. If I hadn't read every article in conventional medical literature and found them dancing around the topic of female hormones, leaving me feeling cheated by the lack of validity in their data and commitment in their results, I wouldn't have started my own research. I did because I had no choice. I had no option but to take it upon myself to formulate a viable, safe, and lasting solution.

This need became the first step in the sequence that led to the program defined in *The Hormone Solution*. I have provided you with the scientific basis and clinical proof that helped me reach this simple yet life-changing conclusion.

The second step was finding the solution. But before I found natural hormones, I had to objectively and seriously address other options available. I have introduced you to the conventional and alternative treatments I evaluated before reaching the natural hormone solution. I thought it important to share this information with you for a few reasons. Most physicians you will be seeing are not yet familiar with natural hormones. So they will offer other options to you. It's important for you to know what these options are, how they work, and what their pitfalls may be. This book is designed to help you make informed decisions. If you choose to try other options, be they conventional or alternative, I urge you to exercise caution and never become a victim in the process. If this is your first exposure to natural hormones, I hope you become a testimonial to their positive benefits.

The decision to use natural hormones must arise from knowledge and strength, not desperation and fear. And finally, I don't want you to work around your doctor when taking them. *The Hormone Solution* has given you the scientific information your doctor needs to feel comfortable prescribing natural hormones and a program you can easily follow under his or her guidance.

"Good solutions are simple solutions," a Nobel Prize–winning professor I had in medical school once taught me. *The Hormone Solution* is a simple solution. Using natural hormones, simple molecules derived from soy and yams, I have created a comprehensive program for the prevention and elimination of symptoms of hormone imbalance at any age. Take the book to your doctor, follow the program, and join me in the natural solution to all symptoms of hormone imbalance.

Available Hormone Preparations

Transdermal Estrogen Patches, Synthetic

Brand Name	Active Ingredient	Strengths (released per 24 hours)
Alora	17beta-estradiol	0.05, 0.075, 0.1 mg twice weekly
Climara	17beta-estradiol	0.025, 0.05, 0.075, 0.1 mg once weekly
FemPatch	17beta-estradiol	0.05, 0.1 mg twice weekly
Menorest	17beta-estradiol	0.0375, 0.05, 0.073 mg twice weekly
Vivelle-Dot/ Vivelle	17beta-estradiol	0.0375, 0.05, 0.075, 0.1 mg twice weekly
Estraderm	17beta-estradiol	0.05, 0.1 mg twice weekly
Esclim	17beta-estradiol	0.025, 0.0375, 0.05, 0.075, 0.1 mg twice weekly
CombiPatch	17beta-estradiol and norethindrone acetate	0.05 mg estradiol and 0.14 mg norethindrone every 3–4 days

Gels, Natural

Brand Name	Active Ingredient	Strengths
Estradiol	Estradiol	1.5 mg gel once a day
Triest gel	10% estrone, 10% estradiol, and 80% estriol	2.5 mg gel once daily 5 mg gel once daily

Oral Estrogen, Natural and Synthetic

Brand Name	Active Ingredient	Strengths
Triestrogen	10% estrone, 10% estradiol, and 80% estriol (natural)	Tablets 1.25 and 2.5 mg twice daily
Biestrogen	20% estradiol, 80% estriol (natural)	Tablets 1.25 and 2.3 mg twice daily
Estrace	Micronized estradiol (natural)	Tablets 0.3, 0.625, 1.25, and 2.5 mg daily
Estinyl	Ethinyl estradiol (synthetic)	Tablets 0.02, 0.05, and 0.5 mg daily
Estratab Menest Cenestin	Estrerified estrogens (synthetic)	Tablets 0.3, 0.625, 1.25, and 2.5 mg daily
Ogen/ Ortho-Est	Estropipate (Estrone sulfate) (synthetic)	Tablets 0.625, 1.25, and 2.5 mg daily
Premarin	Conjugated equine estrogens (synthetic)	Tablets 0.3, 0.625, 0.9, 1.25, and 2.5 mg daily

Vaginal Estrogen Creams, Natural and Synthetic

Brand Name	Active Ingredient	Strengths
Estrace	Micronized estradiol (natural)	Cream 1.0 mg/1 g base
Etriol	Micronized estriol (natural)	Cream 0.5 mg/1 g base
Premarin	Conjugated equine estrogens (synthetic)	Cream 0.625 mg/ 1 g base
Estring	Estradiol (natural)	Ring 2 mg reservoir, change every 90 days
Ogen	Estropipate (synthetic)	Cream 1.5 mg/1 g base
Ortho Dienestrol	Dienestrol (synthetic)	Cream 0.1% dienestrol

Progestins, Synthetic

Brand Name	Active Ingredient	Strengths
Provera	Medroxyprogesterone	Tablets 2.5, 5, and 10 mg
Amen	Medroxyprogesterone	Tablets 10 mg
Cycrin	Medroxyprogesterone	Tablets 2.5, 5, and 10 mg
Micronor	Norethindrone	Tablets 0.35 mg
Norlutin	Norethindrone	Tablets 5 mg
Norlutate	Norethindrone acetate	Tablets 5 mg

Progesterone, Natural

Brand Name	Active Ingredient	Strengths
Oral micronized progesterone	Micronized progesterone	Tablets 50, 100, and 200 mg
Prometrium	Micronized progesterone	Tablets 100 mg
Percutaneous progesterone cream	Micronized progesterone	Cream 5% progesterone
Progesterone gel	Micronized progesterone	Gel 100 or 200 mg

Combined Products, Natural and Synthetic

Brand Name	Active Ingredient	Strengths
Premphase	Conjugated equine estrogens and medroxyprogesterone acetate (synthetic)	Tablets 0.625 mg days 1–14, 0.625 and 5 mg days 15–28
Prempro	Conjugated equine estrogens and medroxyprogesterone acetate (synthetic)	Tablets 0.625 and 2.5 mg daily, 0.625 and 5 mg daily
Triest plus oral micronized progesterone	10% estrone, 10% estradiol, 80% estriol plus 50 to 100 mg micronized progesterone (natural)	Tablets 1.25 mg TriEst plus 50–100 mg oral micronized progesterone twice a day
OrthoPrefest	17beta-estradiol and Norgestimate (synthetic)	Tablets 1 mg 17beta-estradiol daily plus 3-days-on, 3-days-off cycle of 0.09 mg Norgestimate
Femhrt	Ethinyl estradiol and norethindrone acetate (synthetic)	Tablets 0.005 mg ethinyl, estradiol and 1 mg norethindrone acetate
Estratest	Esterified estrogens and methyltestosterone (synthetic)	Tablets 1.25 mg esterified estrogens and 2.5 mg methyltestosterone

Testosterone, Natural and Synthetic

Brand Name	Active Ingredient	Strengths
Oral micronized testosterone	Micronized testosterone (natural)	Tablets 1.25, 2.5, and 5 mg
Methyltestos-terone	Methyltestosterone (synthetic)	Tablets 1.25 and 2.5 mg
Testosterone propionate	Testosterone propionate (synthetic)	Ointment or cream 1–2%
Androgel	Micronized testosterone (natural)	1% unit dose
Androderm	Testosterone anthate salt (synthetic)	5 mg

Glossary of Terms

Alzheimer's disease A degenerative disease of the central nervous system characterized by senility; named for the German physician Alois Alzheimer.

Androgen Any of a number of masculinizing hormones present in the male or female body.

Androstenediol An androgenic (masculinizing) hormone made in the ovaries and adrenals that can be metabolized in fatty tissues into the estrogens—estradiol, estriol, or estrone—or can be converted into testosterone.

Andropause Gradual changes that take place in men as their sex hormone production declines; the male version of the female menopause.

Cervix The narrow outer end of the uterus that protrudes into the vagina.

Corpus luteum The progesterone-secreting tissue mass that forms after ovulation from the ovarian follicle after it has released an egg.

Designer hormones Hormones or hormonelike synthetic pharmaceuticals that are designed to target specific actions in the body.

Endocrine Ductless glands (such as the thyroid and pituitary) or tissue that produce secretions that are carried in the bloodstream.

Endometrium The nutrient-rich mucous membrane lining the uterus.

Estradiol Also known as E_2, the main human estrogen produced in the ovaries.

Estriol Also known as E_3, an estrogen that is a relatively weak metabolite of estradiol; it's produced in larger quantities in the body during pregnancy.

Estrogen The name for the group of substances that have feminizing effects in the body; sex hormones that promote estrus and stimulate female secondary sex characteristics.

Estrone Also known as E_1, the main estrogen produced in the female body after menopause, largely through conversion of androgens in fatty and other tissues.

Fertility In women, the ability to become pregnant; the capability to produce offspring.

Fibroids Areas of fibrous growth in the uterus.

Follicle The area in the ovary where the egg matures before ovulation.

Follicular phase That early phase of the menstrual cycle following menstruation when follicles are growing in the ovary and the egg matures prior to ovulation; also described as the proliferative phase.

FSH (follicle-stimulating hormone) A hormone secreted by the anterior pituitary gland that stimulates development of the ovarian follicles, maturation of the egg, and the production of estrogen.

GnRH (gonadotropin-releasing hormone) A hormone sent by the hypothalamus gland to the pituitary, prompting the release of either FSH or LH (luteinizing hormone).

Gonad Reproductive glands (ovaries or testes).

Hormone A substance produced by cells that circulates in the bloodstream and in body fluids and exerts specific effects on cells elsewhere in the body.

Hot flash A sudden and sometimes prolonged flushing and feeling of heat; it's caused by the rapid dilation of capillaries and is associated with hormone imbalance.

HRT (hormone replacement therapy) The replacement by an outside source of one or more hormones depleted in the body. Refers to synthetic hormones.

Hysterectomy The surgical procedure by which the uterus and cervix are removed. (When the ovaries are also removed, it's called Oophorectomy.)

LH (luteinizing hormone) A hormone secreted by the anterior pituitary gland that prompts ovulation.

Luteal phase The late phase of the menstrual cycle following ovulation when the corpus luteum secretes progesterone.

Mammography An X ray of the breast; used to detect cancer and other abnormalities.

Menarche The first menstrual period experienced in adolescence.

Menopause The normal cessation of the menstrual cycle in women, occurring usually in the late forties and early fifties. Clinically, it's defined as the time after a woman has not had a period for a year.

Menstrual cycle Usually twenty-eight to thirty days in length; the term refers to the changes that take place in a woman's body between two menstrual periods.

Osteoporosis A condition of "brittle bones" that some older women are at risk of developing. It is characterized by reduction in bone density and mass, and an increase in porosity. Osteoporosis leads to a higher risk of fractures.

Ovaries The pair of female reproductive organs on both sides of the pelvis that produce eggs and secrete sex hormones.

Ovulation The release of an egg from the ovarian follicle fourteen days before the beginning of menstruation: the point in time in which fertilization can occur.

Perimenopause A term used to describe the period of time just before menopause; it may last as long as several years.

Phytohormones Hormones found in plants that may exert hormonal effects in the human body.

PMS (premenstrual syndrome) A characterization of a group of symptoms sometimes experienced in the days leading up to menstruation.

Progesterone A female sex hormone secreted by the corpus luteum to prepare for the implantation of an egg into the uterus; during pregnancy, it's also secreted by the placenta in high levels; literally progestational, progesterone is used to balance the effects of estrogen in a hormone supplementation regime.

Progestin A synthetic version of progesterone possessing minimal similarity to the molecular structure of progesterone. Used in synthetic hormone replacement therapy.

Raloxifene A designer estrogen claimed to curb postmenopausal bone loss.

Systemic Affecting the whole body function.

Tamoxifen Designer estrogen that interferes with the action of estrogen specifically on breast tissue.

Testosterone A male sex hormone that is also seen in small quantities in females. In males it is responsible for expression of secondary sexual characteristics. It may be added to hormone supplementation therapy to enhance libido.

Uterus The organ in a woman's body where a fertilized egg is implanted and where the embryo and fetus grows.

Vaginal atrophy Thinning and drying of vaginal wall, which usually occurs during menopausal years.

Resources

Web Sites

www.HormoneSolution.com

www.ErikaSchwartzMD.com

www.naturalwoman.org

www.naturalhormonepharmacy.com

www.nhpinfo.com

www.hormonesnow.com

Organizations

American Menopause Foundation, 350 Fifth Avenue, Suite 2822, New York, NY 10018; (212) 714-2398, Fax (212) 714-1252.

National Women's Health Network, 514 10th Street NW, Suite 400, Washington, DC 20004; (202) 347-1140.

National Menopause Foundation, Center for Climacteric Study, Gainesville, FL 32601; (800) 886-4354.

Natural Woman Institute, 8539 Sunset Boulevard, Los Angeles, CA 90069; (888) 489-6626

Compounding Pharmacies

The Natural Hormone Pharmacy, (800) 522-6692.

Women's International Pharmacy, (800) 279-5708.

Recommended Reading

J. Beasley and J. Swift. *The Kellogg Report: The Impact of Nutrition, Environment, and Lifestyle on the Health of Americans.* Annandale-on-Hudson. The Institute of Health Policy and Practice of the Bard College Center, 1989.

Ellen Brown and Lynn Walker. *Menopause and Estrogen.* Frog, Ltd., 1996.

Robert Butler and Myrna Lewis. *Love and Sex After 60.* Ballantine Books, 1993.

Christine Conrad. *A Woman's Guide to Natural Hormones.* Perigee, 2000.

Laura Corio, MD. *The Change Before the Change.* Bantam, 2001.

R. Cottrell. *Stress Management* (Wellness Series). Dushken, 1992.

William Evans and Irwin Rosenberg. *Biomarkers: The 10 Determinants of Aging You Can Control.* Simon and Schuster, 1992.

Oz Garcia. *Oz Garcia's Healthy High-Tech Body.* Regan Books, 2001.

Donna Howell. *The Unofficial Guide to Coping with Menopause.* Macmillan, 1991.

John Lee, MD. *What Your Doctor May Not Tell You about Menopause.* Warner, 1996.

Christiane Northrup, MD. *The Wisdom of Menopause.* Bantam, 2001.

Susan Rako, MD. *The Hormone of Desire.* Harmony Books, 1996.

Adam Romoff, MD. *Estrogen—How and Why It Can Save Your Life.* Golden Books, 1999.

Barbara Kass-Annese, RNC, NP, MSN. *Management of the Perimenopausal and Postmenopausal Woman: A Total Wellness Program.* Lippincott, 1999.

References

Pharmaceutical Products

Drug Facts and Comparisons 2001. St. Louis: Facts & Comparisons, 2001.

Reproductive Physiology

Speroff L, Glass RH, Kase NG. *Clinical Gynecologic Endocrinology and Infertility*. Baltimore: Williams & Wilkins, 1994.

Greendale G, Judd H. "Menopause." In: Carr, Pet, et al. *The Medical Care of Women*. Philadelphia: WB Saunders, 1995.

Longscope C. "The Endocrinology of the Menopause." In: *Treatment of the Post-Menopausal Woman: Basic and Clinical Aspects*. New York: Raven Press, 1994.

Scott J, et al. *Danforth's Obstetrics and Gynecology*, 7th ed. Philadelphia: JB Lippincott, 1994:774.

Causes and Symptoms of Hormone Imbalance

Arpels JC. "The Female Brain Hypoestrogenic Continuum from the Pre-menstrual Syndrome to Menopause." *Journal of Reproductive Medicine* 41.9 (1996):633–639.

Aronne LJ. "Weight Gain During the Perimenopause." *Menopause Management* (Nov/Dec 1999):6–11.

Asplund R, Aberg H. "Nocturnal Micturition, Sleep and Well-Being in Women of Ages 40–64 Years" *Maturitas* 24 (1996):73–81.

Bachman, David L. "Sleep Disorders with Aging: Evaluation and Treatment." *Geriatrics* 47.9 (1992):53–61.

Bachmann GA, et al. "Female Sexuality During the Menopause." *OBG Management* suppl. 11.5 (1999).

Bales L. "Treatment of the Perimenopausal Female." *Primary Care Update Ob/Gyns* 5.2 (1998):90–94.

Begly S. "Understanding Perimenopause." *Newsweek* Special Edition (spring/summer 1999):34.

Byyny R, Speroff L. *A Clinical Guide for the Care of Older Women: Primary and Preventative Care.* Baltimore: Williams & Wilkins, 1996.

Casper RF, Yen SSC, Wilkes MM. "Menopausal Flushes: A Neuroendocrine Linked with Pulsatile Luteinizing Hormone Secretion." *Science* 205 (1979):823–825.

Dennerstein L, et al. "Sexuality, hormones and the menopausal transition." *Maturitas* 26 (1997):83–93.

Faddy MJ, et al. "Accelerated Disappearance of Ovarian Follicles in Mid-Life: Implications of Forecasting Menopause." *Human Reproduction* 7 (1992):1342.

Greendale GA, Sowers M. "The Menopause Transition." *Endocrinology and Metabolism Clinics of North America* 26.2 (1997):261–276.

Hahn PM, Wong J, Reid RL. "Menopausal-Like Hot Flashes Reported in Women of Reproductive Age." *Fertility and Sterility* 70.5 (1998):913–918.

Harris B, Lovett RG, Newcombe GF, Read R, Riad-Fahmy D. "Maternity Blues and Major Endocrine Changes:

Cardiff Puerperal Mood and Hormone Study II (Wales)." *British Medical Journal* (Apr 9, 1994).

Johnson K. "Low Testosterone May Underlie Inhibited Libido." *Obstetrics/Gynecologic News* 15 (Nov 1998):23.

MacGregor EA. "Menstruation, Sex, Hormones, and Migraine." *Neurologic Clinics* 15.1(1997):125–141.

Schwingl PJ, et al. "Risk Factors for Menopausal Hot Flashes." *Obstetrics and Gynecology* 84 (1994):29.

Sherwin BB. "Estrogen Effects of Cognition in Menopausal Women." *Neurology* 48 suppl. 7 (1997):S21–S26.

Speroff L, Glass RH, Kase NG. *Clinical Gynecologic Endocrinology and Infertility,* 5th ed. Baltimore: Williams & Wilkins, 1994.

Speroff L, et al. "Your Menopausal Patient: Individualizing Management." *Contemporary Ob/Gyn* suppl. (1998):4–25.

Spiegel K, Leproult R, Van Cauter E. "Impact of Sleep Debt in Metabolic and Endocrine Function." *Lancet* 354 (1999):1435–1439.

Stark S. "Migraine in Women." *Female Patient* 24 (1999):53–69.

Washburn SA. "Estradiol and Progesterone Effects on the Central Nervous System." *Menopausal Medicine* 5.4 (1997):5–8.

"Hair Loss in Women." *Mayo Clinic Health Letter* (Feb 1997).

Heart Disease

Baron UM, Galea R, Brincat M. "Carotid Artery Wall Changes in Estrogen-Treated and Untreated

Postmenopausal Women." *Obstetrics and Gynecology* 1 (1998):983.

Barbieri RL, Legro RS, Lewis SJ, Walsh BW, Welty FK, eds. "Managing Hyperlipidemia in Women." *Current Therapeutics* (1999).

Bass KM, et al. "Plasma Lipoprotein Levels As Predictors of Cardiovascular Deaths in Women." *Circulation* 153 (1993):2209.

Bergmann S, Sieger G, Wahrburg U, Schulte H. "Influence of Menopause and Lifestyle Factors on High-Density Lipoproteins in Middle-Aged Women." *Journal of the North American Menopause Society* 4 (1997):52.

Bush TL, Miller VT. "Effects of Pharmacologic Agents Used During Menopause: Impact on Lipids and Lipoproteins." In: Mishell DR Jr, ed. *Menopause: Physiology and Pharmacology.* Chicago: Year Book Medical, 1987:187–208.

Castelli W. "Your Healthy Heart." *Prevention* (Apr 1996):102.

Castelli WP, et al. "Lipids and Risk of Coronary Heart Disease: The Framingham Study." *Annals of Epidemiology* 2 (1992):23–28.

Chen FP, Lee N, Soong YK. "Changes in the Lipoprotein Profile in Postmenopausal Women Receiving Hormone Replacement Therapy: Effects of Natural and Synthetic Progesterone." *Journal of Reproductive Medicine* 43 (1998):568.

Clardson TB. "The Effects of Hormone Replacement Therapy on Key Risk Factors for Cardiovascular Disease." *Hormone Replacement Therapy Cardiovascular Health.* Fairlawn, NJ: MPE Communications, 2000.

Grodstein F, Stampfer MJ. "The Epidemiology of Coronary Heart Disease and Estrogen Replacement in Post-Menopausal Women." *Progress in Cardiovascular Diseases* 18 (1995):199.

Henderson BE, Paganini-Hill A, Ross RK. "Estrogen Replacement and Protection from Acute Myocardial Infarction." *American Journal of Obstetrics and Gynecology* 159 (1998):312.

Herrington DM, et al. "Effects of Estrogen Replacement on the Progression of Coronary-Artery Atherosclerosis." *New England Journal of Medicine* 343 (2000):522.

Lindheim SR, Notelovitz M, Feldman EB, et al. "The Independent Effects of Exercise and Estrogen on Lipids and Lipoproteins in Postmenopausal Women." *Obstetrics and Gynecology* 83 (1994):167.

Newton KM, LaCroix AZ. "Hormone Replacement Therapy and Tertiary Prevention of Coronary Heart Disease." *Menopausal Medicine* 7.2 (1999):5–8.

Simon HB. *Conquering Heart Disease.* New York: Little, Brown, 1994.

Sotelo M, Johnson SR. "The Effects of Hormone Replacement Therapy on Coronary Heart Disease." *Endocrinology and Metabolism Clinics of North America* 26.2 (1997):313–327.

Speroff L. "Postmenopausal Hormone Therapy and Cardiovascular System." Oregon Health Services University School of Medicine, 1997. *Contemporary Ob/Gyn* 42.6.

Speroff L. "The Heart and Estrogen/Progestin Replacement Study (HERS)." *Maturitas* 31 (1998):9.

Sullivan JM, et al. "Estrogen Replacement and Coronary Artery Disease: Effect on Survival in

Postmenopausal Women." *Archives of Internal Medicine* 150 (1990):2557.

Sullivan J, Fowlkes L. "The Clinical Aspects of Estrogen and the Cardiovascular System." *Obstetrics and Gynecology* 87 (1996):368.

Taskinen MR, et al. "Hormone Replacement Therapy Lowers Plasma Lp(a) Concentrations, Comparison Cyclic Transdermal and Continuous Estrogen Progestin Regimens." *Arterioscler Thromb Vasc Biol* 16 (1996):1215–1221.

"Heart Disease Is the Number 1 Killer of Women in the United States." *Heart Strong Woman.* The American College of Obstetricians and Gynecologists, 1998.

Whitcroft SI, Crook D, Marsh MS, et al. "Long Term Effects of Oral and Transdermal Hormone Replacement Therapies on Serum Lipid and Lipoprotein Concentrations." *Obstetrics and Gynecology* 84 (1994):222.

Osteoporosis

Anderson JJ, et al. "Roles of Diet and Physical Activity in the Prevention of Osteoporosis." *Scand Jour Rheumatol* suppl. 103 (1996):65–74.

Cauley JA, Lucas FL, Kuller LH, et al. "Bone Mineral Density and Risk of Breast Cancer in Older Women: The Study of Osteoporotic Fractures." *Journal of the American Medical Association* 276 (1996):1404.

Cauley JA, et al. "Bone Mineral Density and the Risk of Breast Cancer in Older Women: The Study of Osteoporotic Fractures." Study of Osteoporotic Fractures Research Group. *JAMA* 276 (1996):1404–1408.

Consensus Development Conference. "Diagnosis, Prophylaxis, and Treatment of Osteoporosis." *American Journal of Medicine* 94 (1993):64.

DeSouza MJ, Prestwool KM, Luciano AA, Miller BE, Nulsen JC. "A Comparison of the Effect of Synthetic and Micronized Hormone Replacement Therapy on Bone Mineral Density and Biochemical Markers of Bone Metabolism." *Journal of the North American Menopause Society* 3 (1996):140.

Ettinger B, Genant HK, Steiger P, Madvig P. "Low-Dosage Micronized 17B Estradiol Prevents Bone Loss in Postmenopausal Women." *American Journal of Obstetrics and Gynecology* 166 (1992):479.

Hosking D, et al. "Prevention of Bone Loss with Alendornate in Postmenopausal Women Under 60 Years of Age." Early Postmenopausal Intervention Cohort Study Group. *New England Journal of Medicine* 338 (1998):485.

Lindsay R. "Prevention and Treatment of Osteoporosis." *Lancet* 341 (1993):801.

NIH Consensus Development Panel. "Osteoporosis Prevention, Diagnosis, and Therapy." *JAMA* 285 (2001):785.

Ravin P, et al. "Alendronate in Early Postmenopausal Women: Effects on Bone Mass During Long-Term Treatment and After Withdrawal." Alendronate Osteoporosis Prevention Study Group. *Journal of Clinical Endocrinology and Metabolism* 85 (2001):4920.

Zhang Y, et al. "Bone Mass and the Risk of Cancer Among Postmenopausal Women." *New England Journal of Medicine* 336 (1998):611–617.

Hormonal Therapies

Bachmann GA, et al. "Role of Androgens in the Menopause." *OBG Management* suppl. 10.7 (1998):90–94.

Bales L. "Treatment of the Perimenopausal Female." *Primary Care Update OB/Gyns* 5.2 (1998):90–94.

Buyuk E, Gurler A, Emerus M. "Relationship Between Circulating Estradiol Levels, Body Mass Index, and Breakthrough Bleeding in Postmenopausal Women Receiving Hormone Replacement Therapy." *Journal of the North American Menopause Society* 5 (1998):24.

Byyny R, Speroff L. *A Clinical Guide for the Care of Older Women: Primary and Preventative Care,* 2d ed. Baltimore: Williams & Wilkins, 1996.

Coope J. "Hormonal and Non-Hormonal Interventions for Menopausal Symptoms." *Maturitas* 23 (1996):159–168.

Dentali S. "Hormones and Yams; What's the Connection?" *American Heart Association* 10 (1995):4.

Follingstad A. "Estriol, the Forgotten Hormone." *JAMA* 239.1 (1978):29–39.

Henderson VW, et al. "The Epidemiology of Estrogen Replacement Therapy and Alzheimer's Disease." *Neurology* (1997):48.

Lee J. *Natural Progesterone: The Multiple Roles of a Remarkable Hormone.* Sebastopol, CA: BLL Publishing, 1994.

Lobo R. "Benefits and Risks of Estrogen Replacement Therapy." *American Journal of Obstetrics and Gynecology* 173 (1995):982.

Lobo R, et al. "The Menopause Study Group: Metabolic Impact of Adding Medroxyprogesterone Acetate to Conjugated Estrogen Therapy in Post-Menopausal Women." *Obstetrics and Gynecology* 84 (1994):987.

Lobo RA. "The Role of Progestins in Hormone Replacement Therapy." *American Journal of Obstetrics and Gynecology* 166 (1992):1997.

Lourwood DL. "Guide to Hormone Replacement Therapy." *Ob/Gyn* Special Edition (spring 1999):15–20.

Magill PJ. "Investigation of the Efficacy of Progesterone Pessaries in the Relief of Symptoms of Premenstrual Syndrome." *British Journal of General Practice* (Nov 1995):598–593.

Nachtigall LE. "Emerging Delivery Systems for Estrogen Replacement Aspects of Transdermal and Oral Delivery." *American Journal of Obstetrics and Gynecology* 173 (1995):993.

Nilsson K, Kumer G. "Low-Dose Oestradiol in the Treatment of Urogenital Oestrogen Deficiency: A Pharmacokinetic and Pharmacodynamic Study. *Maturitas* 15 (1992):121.

Oregon Health Sciences University School of Medicine. "Advances in Transdermal Postmenopausal Hormone Therapy." *Ob/Gyn* suppl. (Jan 1999).

Rigg LA, Hermann H, Yen SSDC. "Absorption of Estrogens from Vaginal Creams." *New England Journal of Medicine* 298 (1978):195.

Simon JA. "Effects of Progestins and Progesterone on CNS Function." *Menopausal Medicine* 6.4 (1998):8–12.

Weber AA. "Effects of Estrogens and Androgens on the Libido of Women Following Surgical and Natural Menopause." *Menopausal Medicine* 7.1 (1999).

"Women May Prefer Natural Progesterone Over Synthetic." *Mayo Clinic Women's Health Source* 3.8 (1999):3.

Worcester S. "New Progesterones Offer Good Alternatives" *Obstetrics/Gynecologic News* (July 1, 1999):11.

The Writing Group for the PEPI. "Trial Effects of Estrogen or Estrogen/Progestin Regimens on Heart Disease Risk Factors in Postmenopausal Women: The Postmenopausal Estrogen/Progestin Intervention (PEPI) Trial." *JAMA* 273 (1995):199–208.

Skin

Berman RS, et al. "Risk Factors Associated with Women's Compliance with Estrogen Replacement Therapy." *Journal of Women's Health* 6 (1997):219–226.

Pierard GE, et al. "Effect of Hormone Replacement Therapy for Menopause on the Mechanical Properties of the Skin." *American Geriatric Society* 43 (1995):662–665.

Roxenberg S, et al. "Compliance to Hormone Replacement Therapy." *Int Jour Fertil Menopausal Stud* 40 (1995):S23–32.

Vaillant L, Callens A. "Hormone Replacement Treatment: A Skin Aging Therapy." *American Geriatric Society* 51 (1996):67–70.

Alternative Medicine

Albertazzi P, Pansini F, Bonaaccorsi G, Zanotti L, de Aloysio E, de Aloysio D. "The Effect of Dietary Soy Supplementation on Hot Flushes" *Obstetrics and Gynecology* 91.1 (1998):6–11.

Brody JE. "Americans Gamble on Herbs as Medicine." *New York Times* (Feb 9, 1999):F1, F7.

Elgharmy MI, Shihata IM. "Biological Activity of Phytoestrogens." *Planta Medica* 13 (1965):352–357.

Goldberg B. *Alternative Medicine Guide to Women's Health,* vol. 1. Tiburon, CA: Future Medicine Publishing, 1998:220–229.

Kass-Annese B. "Alternative Therapies for Menopause." *Clinical Obstetrics and Gynecology* 43.1 (2000):162–183.

Norman T, Setchell K, Bingham S. "Hormonal Effects of Soy." *American Journal of Clinical Nutrition* suppl. 68 (1998):1531S–1533S.

Taylor M. "Alternatives to Conventional HRT: Phytoestrogens and Botanicals." *Contemporary Ob/Gyn* (June 1999):27–50.

Designer Estrogens

Adler S, Sadovsky Y. "Selective Modulation of Estrogen Receptor Action." *Journal of Clinical Endocrinology and Metabolism* 83 (1998):3.

Berliere M, Charles A, Galant C, Donnez J. "Uterine Side of Tamoxifen: A Need for Systematic Pretreatment Screening." *Obstetrics and Gynecology* 91 (1998):40.

Cheng WF, Lin HH, Torng OL, Huang SC. "Comparison of Endometrial Changes Among Symptomatic Tamoxifen-Treated and Nontreated Premenopausal and Postmenopausal Breast Cancer Patients." *Gynecologic Oncology* 66 (1997):233.

Cohen I, Altaras MM, Beyth Y, et al. "Estrogen and Progesterone Receptors in the Endometrium of Postmenopausal Breast Cancer Patients Treated with Tamoxifen and Progestogens." *Gynecologic Oncology* 66 (1997):83.

Cohen I, Rosen DJD, Shapira J, et al. "Endometrial Changes with Tamoxifen: Comparison Between Tamoxifen-Treated and Nontreated Asymptomatic, Post-

Menopausal Breast Cancer Patients." *Gynecologic Oncology* 52 (1994):185.

Daniel Y, Inbar M, Bar-Am A, Peyser MR, Lessing JB. "The Effects of Tamoxifen Treatment on the Endometrium." *Fertility-Sterility* 65 (1996):1085.

Delmas PD, Bjarnson NH, Mitlak BH, et al. "Effects of Raloxifene on Bone Mineral Density, Serum Cholesterol Concentrations, and Uterine Endometrium in Post-menopausal Women." *New England Journal of Medicine* 337 (1997):1641.

Fisher B, Constantino JP, Redmond CK, Fisher ER, Wickerman DL, Cronin WM, et al. "Endometrial Cancer in Tamoxifen-Treated Breast Cancer Patients: Findings from the National Surgical Adjuvant Breast and Bowel Project B-14." *Journal of the National Cancer Institute* 86 (1994):527.

Gusberg SB. "Tamoxifen for Breast Cancer Associated Endometrial Cancer." *Cancer* (Apr 1990):1464.

Heaney RP, Draper MW. "Raloxifene and Estrogen: Comparative Bone-Remodeling Kinetics." *Journal of Clinical Endocrinology and Metabolism* 82 (1997):3425.

Henigh RM. "Behind the Buzz on Designer Estrogens, Questions Linger." *New York Times* (June 21, 1998).

Nayfield SG, Gorin MB. "Tamoxifen-Associated Eye Disease: A Review." *Journal of Clinical Oncology* 14 (1996):1018.

Nevan P., Vergote I. "Should Tamoxifen Users Be Screened for Endometrial Lesions?" *Lancet* 351 (1998):155.

Penotti M, Sirone L, Miglierina L, et al. "The Effect of Tamoxifen and Transdermal Estrakiol on Cerebral Arterial Vessels: A Randomized Controlled Study." *American Journal of Obstetrics and Gynecology* 178 (1998):801.

Powles T, Eeles R, Ashley S, et al. "Interim Analysis of the Incidence of Breast Cancer in the Royal Marsden Hospital Tamoxifen Randomized Chemo Prevention Trial." *Lancet* 352 (1998):98.

Pritchard KI. "Is Tamoxifen Effective in Prevention of Breast Cancer?" *Lancet* 352 (1998)

Synthetic Estrogen and Cancer

Bonnier P, Romain S, Giaclolone L, et al. "Clinical and Biologic Prognostic Factors in Breast Cancer Diagnosed During Postmenopausal Hormone Replacement Therapy." *Obstetrics and Gynecology* 85 (1997):11.

Burke W, Lacroix AZ. "Breast Cancer and Hormone Replacement Therapy." *Lancet* 350 (1997):1042.

Bush TL, et al. "Cardiovascular Mortality and Noncontraceptive Use of Estrogen in Women: Results from the Lipid Research Clinics Program Follow-up Study." *Circulation* 75 (1987):1102.

Colditz GA, Hankinson SE, Hunter DJ, et al. "Use of Estrogens and Progestins and the Risk of Breast Cancer in Postmenopausal Women." *New England Journal of Medicine* 332 (1995):1589–93.

DeMott K. "HRT May Increase the Rate of Breast Cancer." *Obstetrics/Gynecologic News* 6 (Jan 1998).

Henderson BE, Paganini-Hill A, Ross RK. "Decreased Mortality in Users of Estrogen Replacement Therapy." *Archives of Internal Medicine* 151 (1991):75.

Nugent P, O'Connell TX. "Breast Cancer and Pregnancy." *Archives of Surgery* 120 (1985):1221.

O'Meara ES, Rossing MA, Daling JR, Elmore JG, Barlow WE, Weiss NS. "Hormone Replacement Therapy

After a Diagnosis of Breast Cancer in Relation to Recurrence and Mortality." *Journal of the National Cancer Institute* 93 (2001):10.

Palmer JR, Rosenberg L, Clarke EA, Miller DR, Shapiro S. "Breast Cancer Risk After Estrogen Replacement Therapy: Results from the Toronto Breast Cancer Study." *American Journal of Epidemiology* 134 (1991):1386–95.

Santen RJ, et al. "Clinical Risk of Breast Cancer with Progestins and in Combination with Estrogen As Hormone Replacement Therapy." *Journal of Clinical Endocrinology and Metabolism* 86 (2001):16.

Schairer C, Byrne C, Keyl PM, et al. "Menopausal Estrogen and Estrogen-Progestin Replacement Therapy and Risk of Breast Cancer." *Cancer Causes Control* 5 (1994):491–500.

Schairer C, et al. "Estrogen Replacement Therapy and Breast Cancer Survival in a Large Screening Study." *Journal of the National Cancer Institute* 91 (1999):264.

Speroff L. "Postmenopausal Hormone Therapy and Breast Cancer." *Obstetrics and Gynecology* 87 (1996):445.

Speroff L. "Postmenopausal Hormone Therapy and Breast Cancer." Oregon Health Sciences University School of Medicine, 1997. *Contemporary Ob/Gyn* 42:1.

Standford JL, Weiss NS, Voight LF, et al. "Combined Estrogen and Progestin Hormone Replacement Therapy in Relation to Risk of Breast Cancer in Middle-Aged Women." *JAMA* 274 (1995):137–42.

Stearns V, et al. "A Pilot Trial Assessing the Efficacy of Paroxetine Hydrochloride (Paxil) in Controlling Hot Flashes in Breast Cancer Survivors." *Annals of Oncology* 11 (2000):17.

Weiss NS, Beresford SAA, Voigt LF, McKnight B. "Estrogen-Progestin Replacement Therapy and Endometrial Cancer." *Journal of the National Cancer Institute* 90 (1998):164.

Diet, Exercise, Lifestyle

Brody JE. "New Look at Dieting: Fat Can Be a Friend." *New York Times* (May 25, 1999):F1, F9.

Cagnacci A, et al. "Effects of Low Doses of Transdermal Estradiol on Carbohydrate Metabolism in Postmenopausal Women." *Journal of Clinical Endocrinology and Metabolism* 74 (1996):1396.

"Disease-Fighting Foods?" *Consumers Reports on Health* (Mar 1998):8–19.

Fine JT, Colditz GA, Coakley EH, Moseley G, Manson JE, Willett WC, Kawachi I. "A Prospective Study of Weight Change and Health-Related Quality of Life in Women." *JAMA* 282 (1999):2136–2142.

Greenwood S. "Fats in the Diet—Helping Midlife Women Make Healthy Choices." *Menopause Management* (May/June 1999):20–24.

Groff JL, Gropp S. *Advanced Nutrition and Human Metabolism.* Belmont, CA: Wadsworth, 2000:147, 252, 449.

Sleep

Polo-Kantola P, Erkkola R, Helenius H, Irjala K, Polo O. "When Does Replacement Therapy Improve Sleep Quality?" *American Journal of Obstetrics and Gynecology* 178 (1998):1002.

Woodward S. "Sleep and Menopause." *The Female Patient* 26 (May 2001):51.

Men and Testosterone

Allan C. "Testosterone Implants Prove Effective." *Internal Medicine World Report* 16 (Jan 2001):1.

Baulieu E-E, Thomas G, Legrain S, et al. "Dehydroepiandrosterone, DHEA Sulfate, and Aging: Contribution of the DHEA Age Study to a Sociobiomedical Issue." *Proc Natl Acad Sci USA* 97 (2000):4279–4284.

Jain P, et al. "Testosterone Supplementation Effective in Some Cases of Erectile Dysfunction." *Journal of Urology* 164 (2000):371–375.

Morley J. "Andropause, Testosterone Therapy, and Quality of Life in Aging Men." *Cleveland Clinic Journal of Medicine* 67 (Dec 2000).

Rostler S. "Satisfied Men Live Longer." *American Journal of Epidemiology* 152 (2000):983–991.

Shifren JL, Braunstein GD, Simon JA, et al. "Transdermal Testosterone Treatment in Women with Impaired Sexual Function After Oophorectomy." *New England Journal of Medicine* 3.43 (2000):682–688.

Tenover JL. "Testosterone Replacement Therapy in Older Adult Men." *Int J Androl* 22 (1999):300–306.

Wang C, Berman N, Longstreth JA, et al. "Pharmacokinetics of Transdermal Testosterone Gel in Hypogonadal Men: Application of Gel at One Site Versus Four Sites: A General Clinical Research Center Study." *Journal of Clinical Endocrinology and Metabolism* 85 (2000):964–969.

General

Barbarch L. "Loss of Sexual Desire." *Menopause Management* 7 (1998):10.

Polo-Kantola P, Erkkola R, Helenius H, Irjala K, Polo O. "When Does Replacement Therapy Improve Sleep Quality?" *American Journal of Obstetrics and Gynecology* 178 (1998):1002.

Schneider LS, Farlow MR, Henderson VW, Pogoda JM. "Effects of Estrogen Replacement Therapy on Response to Tacrine in Patients with Alzheimer's Disease." *Neurology* 46 (1996):1580.

Sherwin BB. "Estrogen, the Brain and Memory." *Journal of the North American Menopause Society* 3 (1996):97.

Sherwin BB. "Estrogen Effects on Cognition in Menopausal Women." *Neurology* 48 (1997):S21.

U.S. Bureau of the Census. "Projections of the Population of the United States: 1977 to 2050." *Current Population Reports* Series P-25, No. 704.

Index